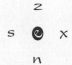

Zen Sex

the way of making love

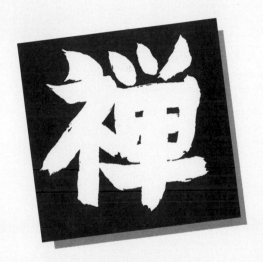

philip toshio sudo

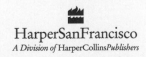

HarperSanFrancisco
A Division of HarperCollins*Publishers*

FIRST HARPERCOLLINS PAPERBACK EDITION PUBLISHED IN 2005
Designed by Philip Toshio Sudo

Library of Congress Cataloging-in-Publication Data
Sudo, Philip Toshio.
Zen Sex : the way of making love / Philip Toshio Sudo. — 1st ed.
p. cm.
Includes bibliographical references.
ISBN 0–06–075799–X (pbk.)
1. Sex instruction—Religious aspects—Zen Buddhism.
2. Sex—Religious aspects—Zen Buddhism. I. Title.
HQ64.S83   2000
613.9'6—dc21   00–020599
05 06 07 08 09 RRD(H) 10 9 8 7 6 5 4 3 2 1

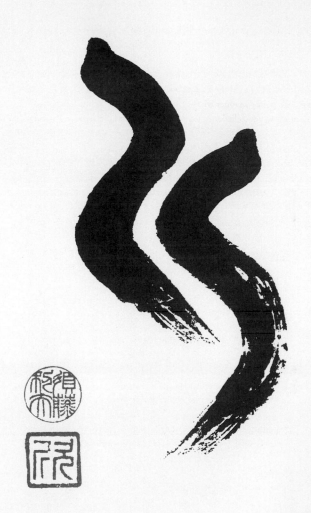

contents

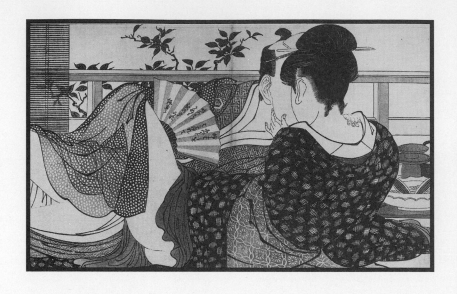

To Tracy

and our miracles,

Naomi

Keith

Jonathan

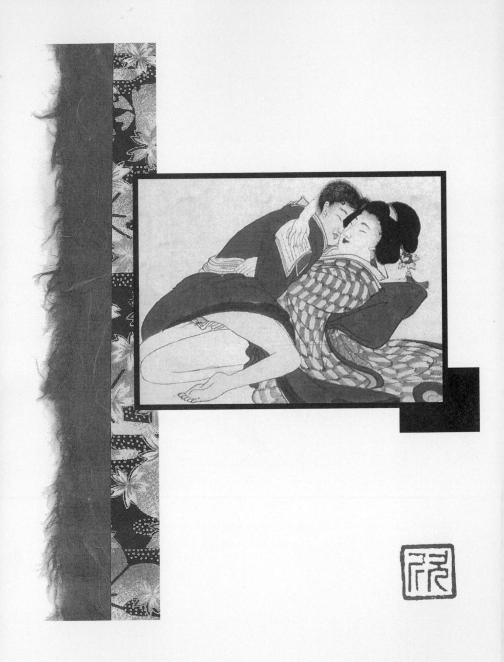

what is zen sex?

A sex-loving monk, you object!
Hot-blooded and passionate, totally aroused.
—Zen master Ikkyu Sojun (1394–1481)

In life, there are many paths to attaining true wisdom. Zen is one of them. Sex is another.

This is where the two paths converge.

On first hearing the term *Zen Sex,* many readers may wonder what could possibly be zen about sex. Zen is supposed to be quiet, tranquil, still as a rock garden. Imagine: *Minimalist sex! Making love without moving!* Sounds like a real turn-on. . . .

And aren't zen monks supposed to be celibate? They take strict ascetic vows. Technically, can there even be Zen Sex?

This book explains that Zen Sex does exist, and it's more

than minimal—in fact, it's mind-blowing. For those who want the truth, *Zen Sex is the best sex you can possibly have.*

How to get it, and what it can mean for your life, is what this book is all about.

We live in an age obsessed with sex. From news accounts of politicians' sex lives to Internet pornography to Viagra to sexual harassment to the latest perversity on "trash TV" talk shows, we're inundated with sexual messages and imagery. Sex has been politicized, criminalized, sensationalized, sold as entertainment—even, in the AIDS crisis, equated with death. Confusing messages abound: Sex is immoral. Sex is dirty. Sex is dangerous. Sex is supposed to be superorgasmic or something's wrong with you, and this magazine/product/lifestyle will correct it.

Lost amid this blather is a simple truth:

Sex is sacred.

For all our obsession with sex—who's getting it, how often, how good—we forget sometimes that sex connects us in the most basic way to the source of Creation. All of us began as a combination of sperm and egg, man and woman. At its best, sex takes us back to that beginning, transcending the mere fulfillment of our animal desires to reveal our inherent divinity as

Creators; it becomes a spiritual endeavor, as profound as any religious rite or ritual, each act symbolizing the origin of life.

Like sex, the study of zen takes us back to our origins as well. It says we can awaken to the divine source at the core of our being, the source from which all things are born, and in so doing, transcend the limits of space and time.

The ideas of zen date back thousands of years, with origins in India and China. Although often considered synonymous with Zen Buddhism, "pure" zen is not a religion, but a spiritual philosophy. The word *zen* itself is Japanese and means "meditation" or "absorption." Traditional zen practice emphasizes sustained meditative breathing, but in the largest sense, zen is simply an absorption in life—the *essence* of life. Quietude and meditation may be aspects of zen, but zen itself is vibrantly alive. Its way is the way of nature, changing like the seasons.

Zen

To say that zen has nothing to do with sex would be to say that sex is unnatural. Nothing could be further from the truth. The way of zen is to allow nature to express itself through all of our actions, whatever they are, in the same way the cherry blossom blooms naturally in the spring.

Religious adherents sometimes renounce sex as an earthly desire to be transcended, and zen monks are no different.

These monks, typically Zen Buddhists, have formalized an approach to zen using a Buddhist system of strictures and rules. Entering the monastery, they take strict vows of asceticism as a means to self-purification. But "pure" zen decries attachment to religious orthodoxy or any doctrinaire pursuit of enlightenment. One of the most revered zen masters in history, Ikkyu Sojun (1394–1481), mocked the rules of monasteries and their extremes of self-denial. In poem after poem, he sang the praises of wine and physical love, of taking a lover and frequenting brothels. A famous example of his poetry follows:

Ten days
In the monastery
Made me restless.
The red thread
On my feet
Is long and unbroken.
If one day you come
Looking for me,
Ask for me
At the fishmonger's,
In the tavern,
Or in the brothel.

To Ikkyu, cutting off relations between men and women so as to attain enlightenment made no sense. In his philosophy of "red thread zen," sex deepened the experience of enlightenment. No one can enter this world without being born of both a man and a woman, he said; we are connected to sex by the "red thread" of blood at birth. Back and back the red thread goes, long and unbroken, to the origin of all being. We're *of* sex. That fact should be embraced, not avoided, Ikkyu said. He openly wore his priest's robes to the pleasure quarters to signify the spiritual nature of his activity:

Me, I am praised as a general of Zen,
Tasting life and enjoying sex to the fullest!

Every moment, be it in sex or quiet meditation, offers a chance for zen realization. Let anything and everything be your source of absorption, for zen truth applies to all things at all times. No matter how you come to zen—through archery, motorcycle maintenance, flower arranging, martial arts, guitar playing, or lovemaking—the progression toward enlightenment is the same. In Ikkyu's words,

Many paths lead from
The foot of the mountain

But at the peak
We all gaze at the
Single bright moon.

Just awaken to the truth; how and where do not matter. Sex offers the same opportunity for enlightenment as anything else.

So many of us go through life searching for sex, bored with sex, ashamed of sex, addicted to sex—whatever—never realizing our potential to awaken and change. But if we apply the principles of zen philosophy to lovemaking, we come to understand the possibilities of spiritual sex—the potential for a transcendent communion to take place. Through this communion, the eternal principles that govern the universe and our lives within it reveal themselves. We come face-to-face with Ikkyu's truth and see its daily workings inside the bedroom and out. In this way, Zen Sex gives life its very meaning.

Be warned, this book is not a modern-day Kama Sutra. It will not teach you ancient love secrets or exercises; it will not detail sexual techniques to drive your lover wild in bed. It does not advocate an "anything goes" or "do whatever gives you pleasure" approach, nor does it suggest conservatism in your sexual frequency or behavior. Whether you make love twice a month or twice a day is up to you. Because Zen Sex is simply this: "Ordinary" sex—*but done with zen awareness.* As the legendary master Rinzai (780–866) put it, true zen is earthy, natural, and nothing special: "Shit and piss, wear your clothes, eat your meals, and in all things be ordinary."

Do not think there is anything wrong with being ordinary. Quite the contrary. If we look deeply enough into the ordinary, as zen prescribes, we discover something extraordinary. This life we've been given, this love within us, our capacity for feeling ecstasy and giving joy—these are nothing short of divine. The problem is, too often we take it all for granted. Life can seem so "ordinary" that our senses become dulled. We keep looking for some extra zip to our lives, some glass of champagne, when all around is pure drinking water. Coursing through every living thing is a vibrant energy, by its very nature a sexual life force. We're all born of it; we all manifest it. The more acutely we become attuned to this "ordinary" energy, the more we begin to marvel at its dimension and wonder, the more we feel it and express it in our lives and lovemaking.

The challenge of zen is to become so absorbed that we feel this energy at every moment. In zen thinking, anything can be the source of meditation, a chance to lose oneself in absorption, whether praying or, as Ikkyu preferred, frolicking in bed with your lover. As he wrote,

The autumn breeze of a single night of love is better than
a hundred thousand years of sterile sitting meditation.

Thus, what makes Zen Sex mind-blowing is not its promise to deliver a superorgasm, but its potential to rescramble our brains—to change the way we look at ourselves, our lovemaking, and the world. What makes it the best sex we can possibly have is not its capacity to fulfill our fantasies, but rather its ability to so deeply absorb us that all thinking is forgotten and we feel the perfection of Divine Love.

We arrive at this truth through the Way of Making Love. The Way of Making Love takes the same transcendent principles that apply to all zen arts and applies them to sex. The Way is available to anyone—man or woman, young or old, married or single, gay or straight. It does not require a lifelong partner. It can take place anywhere, anytime, with anyone, because zen truth is available at all times, for any person willing to practice. Realizing that truth is strictly up to the individual: You.

No words can teach you how to make love; they can only guide you. The actual learning will be up to you, for Zen Sex is all in the doing. As the zen saying goes, "Paths cannot be taught, they can only be taken."

For the purposes of this book, the Way of Making Love is organized into three sections: mind, body, and spirit. Each can be identified by its own symbol—the geometric shapes of the square, triangle, and circle. The use of those shapes is based on a classic painting by the zen master Sengai Gibon (1751–1837), whose primordial *Circle, Triangle, Square* evokes the eternal mystery of zen. Although Sengai never explained the meaning of his painting, *Zen Sex* employs his symbology to represent the three aspects of the Way of Making Love.

The mind is denoted by a square, which represents the box from which our thinking needs to escape.

The body is denoted by a triangle, which represents the temple of our physical form.

The spirit is denoted by a circle, which represents its all-encompassing nature, with no beginning and no end.

Do not be mistaken, though. What applies to one applies equally to the others, for there are no divisions in the Way. To be truly absorbed in lovemaking, the whole of you must be present.

Just make love in the fullest sense of those words, feeling the Power of Love in all its glory. Then, when you've achieved sweet release, you can lie back in bliss on this spinning globe, breathing deeply, and from the core of your being whisper in your lover's ear:

I felt the earth move.

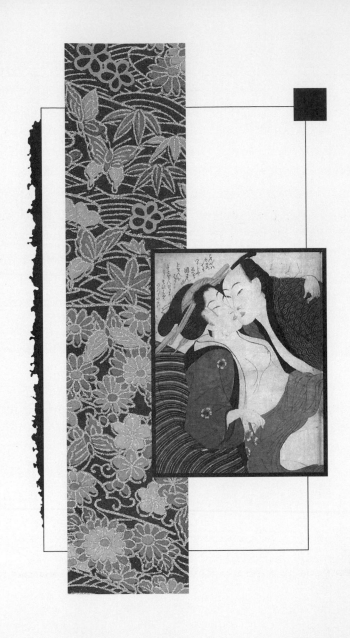

the seven ways of the mind

The ways of proclaiming the Mind all vary, but the same heavenly truth can be seen in each and every one.

—Ikkyu

the ways of Desire
Fantasy
Discovery
Initiating
Anticipation
Surprise
The Familiar

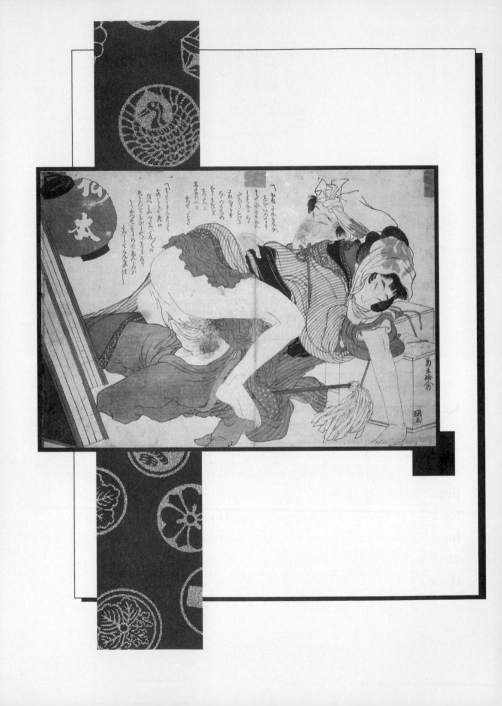

the way of desire

this lust my ceaseless koan
—Ikkyu

In formal zen training, one of the central techniques used to help students discover their true nature is the study of koans. Koans are paradoxical stories or questions that point to the nature of ultimate reality. The most famous koan asks students to contemplate, "What is the sound of one hand clapping?" There is no way to answer the question logically. It forces students to transcend the limits of thinking until they break through to a higher level of understanding. A single koan can be an endless source of revelation, peeling away deeper layers of truth en route to greater and greater awareness.

For Ikkyu, the Way of Desire served as his koan. "When one is thirsty, one dreams of water; when one is cold, one dreams of fire," he says. "I dream of a girl's boudoir; that's my nature." Defying the strictures of the day, he sought to transcend institutional zen and discover truth in the real world of bars and pleasure quarters:

Koan

> *those old koans—meaningless, just ways of*
> * faking virtue*
> *this gorgeous young whore wears silk robes*
> * that hang open about an inch*

There, in that inch, lay his koan.

To Ikkyu, the sight of a beautiful courtesan, her kimono open suggestively, could lead to a meditation as profound as the sound of one hand clapping: *What is the source of this arousal? Why do I have sexual desires? How does lust reveal the ultimate truth?* In Ikkyu's zen, the more we dig into those questions, the closer we come to knowing the divine energy that manifests all things and every action.

According to zen legend, Ikkyu first achieved enlightenment upon hearing the piercing caw of a crow. In succeeding years, as he began to engage in sex and mingle in the "ordinary" world, he wrote,

the crow's caw was ok but one night with a lovely whore
opened a wisdom deeper than what that bird said

To this day, Ikkyu's refusal to renounce sex remains controversial. The strictures of monastic zen forbid "being unchaste," and the Buddha himself taught that enlightenment required celibacy. The Buddha warned that those who succumbed to desire risked being reborn in hell. But Ikkyu believed that even the Buddha's rules were meant to be transcended. "Who needs the Buddhism of ossified masters?" he asked. Once, after eating a meal of fresh octopus (forbidden by zen rules), he remarked, "The taste of the sea, just divine! Sorry, Buddha, this is another precept I just cannot keep." He rejected conformity of any sort, and heaped scorn upon those who believed in a "zen by numbers" approach to enlightenment:

Follow the rule of celibacy blindly and you are no more
*   than an ass.*
Break it and you are only human.
The spirit of zen is manifest in ways as countless as the
*   sands of the Ganges.*
Every newborn is a fruit of the conjugal bond.
For how many eons have the secret blossoms been
*   budding and fading?*

With a young beauty, I am engrossed in fervent love-
play;
We sit in the pavilion, a pleasure girl and this zen monk.
I am enraptured by hugs and kisses
And certainly do not feel as if I am burning in hell.

For all his fervent love-play, Ikkyu understood the dangers of
desire. By flouting the rules of his monastery, he risked veering
into self-indulgence; he knew that a single false step on the
path of zen could lead to a long diversion. Yet he accepted that
risk. "Anybody can enter Buddha's world," he said. "So few can
step into the Devil's." By that he meant, enlightenment is available to all, but to achieve enlightenment *and maintain it in the*
world of desires is vastly difficult. One has to remain committed
to zen above all else and know the difference between partak-
ing of something and indulging in it.

Ikkyu accepted that challenge because he believed human
desires could never be fully extinguished. "I have to admit my
passion never leaves," he said. "Fire is the master, young grasses
appear each spring." Thus, he advocated becoming absorbed
in one's desire, rather than letting it control one's behavior. If
we allow desire to control us, we end up acting out of igno-
rance, selfishness, and egotism, never content with what we
have or who we are. But we can control desire by understand-

ing it, knowing its essence. Therein lies the route to wisdom and happiness. As the classic text of Eastern philosophy, the *Tao Te Ching*, says, "Only those who know when enough is enough will ever have enough."

What is your desire? To be loved? To have a more sizzling sex life? The important thing is to identify it and admit to it. Do not underestimate the bravery required in such an admission. The world is filled with lonely, closed-off souls who can't admit they want love. They sit cloistered in their bedrooms, fearful of rejection, feeling unworthy perhaps, or convinced there is no one out there for them. They wither in stale marriages. They always have an excuse for why they can't step forward. Only a shattering event or the dogged work of a committed evangelist can crack open the hard shell around them.

You, on the other hand, have begun a process of exploration. By admitting that you have desires, you've stepped onto the path of growth. Now the journey begins—a journey that leads ever more deeply inward.

Many people think that having desires implies that something is missing, that there is a hole inside needing to be filled by something "out there." In countless ways, we look "out there" for happiness—for the white knight to ride up and make our lives better, for the people around us to make changes that will satisfy us.

Zen says to stop looking "out there" for the answer. The answer is not "out there"; it is *in here*. Inward is where the key to happiness lies—the key to better sex, to the very meaning of life. There is no need to look anywhere else.

When the monk asked, "What is the path?" the master Nansen replied, "Everyday life is the path." Focus on the *experience* of life, the *experience* of sex, and you may realize that what you think you desire you already have.

If all we longed for was sexual release, we could easily satisfy that through masturbation. But we want more—companionship, affection, a wild romp in the bedroom. Until we grapple with what causes us to look "out there" for happiness, our inner hunger will never be satisfied.

In zen, we *have* the thing we truly lust for. We're *of* it, like every man and woman "born of the conjugal bond" on the planet. We need only awaken to that fact. If you're looking for some extra zest to life, some "super-aliveness" through enlightenment or Zen Sex, it's not there. You can't be more alive than you are—but you can awaken to what living *is*.

Once we understand that we're of the very thing we're looking for, we begin the process of controlling our desires. We begin to "desire without desiring." Let your sex life result naturally from the way you live your life. Don't make sex a goal: "I have to get laid tonight"; "I have to reach climax"; "I have to give my partner a multiple orgasm." Otherwise desire will dominate your behavior. Just live life passionately, make love passionately, absorbed in what you're doing. Don't *try* to do it. *Do* it. The Chinese call this principle *wu wei*: "Doing without 'doing.'" The *Tao Te Ching* describes *wu wei* as the ultimate path of wisdom:

> *The Way does not get closer by searching farther.*
>
> *Therefore,*
> *The sage keeps to the beginning to discover the end.*
> *And finds without seeking;*
> *Arrives without leaving;*
> *Does without doing;*
> *And knows without understanding.*

On the surface, *wu wei* sounds like one of those inscrutable Eastern concepts that make no sense. But zen truth lies beyond the limits of words, often in the middle of a contradiction. When we say something like, "The more things change, the more they stay the same," we know the words work at cross-purposes. Yet we also know the underlying truth of the phrase because we've experienced it. Zen is the same way.

Many men, for example, are said to suffer from a "virgin-whore complex," in which they desire a lover who is sexually both experienced and inexperienced at the same time. Conversely, many women say they want a sensitive, caring man, yet find themselves attracted to the "bad boy" with an edge of danger. Confusion reigns on both sides. How can one person satisfy conflicting desires?

Those who understand *wu wei* know there is a way to be virginal without being a virgin, a way to be whorish without being a whore, a way to be dangerous and safe all at once. We all have different facets to our character, some of them compartmentalized, some of them at odds. There's the person we are at work, the person we are with family, the person we are in the bedroom. Zen Sex says make love with the *whole* of yourself. Bring your innocence *and* experience to the bedroom. Be pure of heart and lust for your lover. Hold out the promise of thrills—and the comfort of safety, all at once. Don't try; just do.

Sexual arousal should arise spontaneously, out of our true nature, in the same way a flower blooms or a fruit falls from the tree when it is ripe. This is zen—arousal without thought of "arousal," desire without "desiring."

The great challenge of zen is to do what comes naturally in every moment; to express our true nature in every action; to

20   *zen sex*

live life aware of both the cosmic order and the tiniest detail. If desire should arise, then follow desire as a means to knowing the truth; its fulfillment should be a spiritual quest. Stay ever-present in the moment, fully absorbed, and the Way of Desire will lead you to Zen Sex.

When it does, lose yourself in meditation over your lover. For in the end, as Ikkyu says,

Only one koan matters
You

the way to zen sex

ask yourself:
what gives me sexual desire?

how deep does your answer go?

z

s ☯ x

n

desire 23

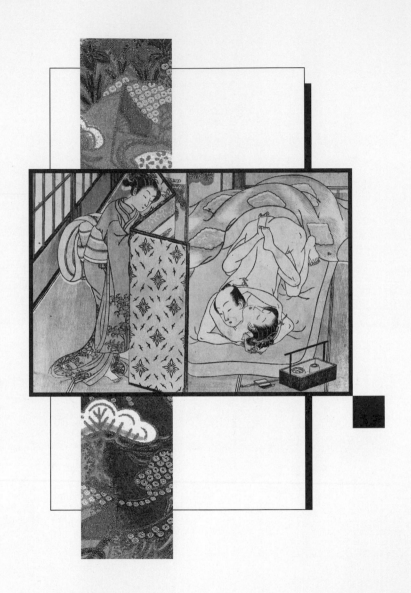

the way of fantasy

I dreamed I was a butterfly dreaming I was a man.
—Chuang-tzu (369–286 B.C.)

There is no better aphrodisiac than what our mind can produce in a flight of fantasy. The merest signal—a picture in a magazine, the sound of a voice on the phone, an absent-minded gaze out the window—can produce an erotically charged inner movie reel, with us as the only audience to please. *The girl listening to the poet bursting with poems thinks nothing*, says Ikkyu, *but he thinks he wants her leaning on the gate while she just listens.* Whomever we want, however we want it, is ours to play out in the mind.

Erotic fantasies are a waking dream, serving up clues to our individual psyches, allowing us to explore our sexuality. They stem from the very source of our creativity—the imagination—linking our conscious and subconscious worlds. By definition, fantasies aren't "real." But the Way of Fantasy is to understand the interplay between reality and imagination, the conscious and the subconscious. To emphasize that idea, Ikkyu often signed his love poems using the pseudonym Mokei, meaning "Dream Boudoir." In zen, the path to the truth lies between the levels of fantasy and reality.

Zen masters teach that this world of time and space—what we call reality—is an illusory veil masking the source of a timeless, spaceless eternity. In the words of the Buddha,

All composite things
Are like a dream, a fantasy, a bubble, and a shadow
Are like a dewdrop and a flash of lightning
They are thus to be regarded.

The challenge is to see that illusion while living in the sensory world of sexual pleasure. When a zen master asked his student, "Does this stick exist or not?" the student replied, "Everything is an objectification of the mind, so no, it does not exist." The master whacked him on the head with it. "Then what just hit your head?" he said. The message: We live in the philosophical realm and the bodily realm at the same time. As the zen saying goes, "Things are not as they seem, nor are they otherwise."

Sexual fantasies put us in touch with this truth, tapping into the same energy that animates the Great Illusion of reality. When we fantasize, we're both participants and observers at the same time, inside of our bodies and yet outside of them in mind. The Way of Fantasy is to see the illusion within the illusion, the movie within the movie, aware of the underlying force that projects the fantasy.

All fantasy originates from the same source, and thus reveals a universal truth. We may be the stars of our own sexual fantasies, imagining ravenous lovers tearing our clothes off, but ultimately, there is no "I" doing the imagining. We who fantasize are merely outlets for the unseen energy of life that plays itself out through us. On the deepest level, we're nothing more than apparitions ourselves, dreamers dreaming within a dream. This feeling was captured in a poetic exchange between the zen master Ryokan (1758–1831) and the love of his life, the nun Teishin (1798–1872). Teishin wrote,

Was it really you
I saw,

Or is this joy
I still feel
Only a dream?

Ryokan answered,

In this dream world
We doze
And talk of dreams—
Dream, dream on,
As much as you wish.

Sexual fantasies allow us to play with this idea of living a dream within a dream. For at the heart of most fantasies is an erotic tension, a delicious pull between seeming opposites: Freedom and the forbidden. Abandon and inhibition. Power and submission. Exploration and safety. Fantasy and reality. The Way of Fantasy is to meditate on that tension and harness the energy created when these opposites interplay. Just read through the following list of common sexual fantasies and you can feel that energy ignite within you.

Common Sexual Fantasies
Having sex with someone in the office

Having sex in an elevator

Having sex with a salesperson or repair person visiting the house

Sex between a teacher and student

Sex between a doctor (or nurse) and patient

Having sex in a public place

Having sex with more than one or a multitude of partners

Having sex in a place in which there is a risk of getting caught

Having sex out in nature

Being sexually taken, possessed, or dominated

Being in complete sexual control of a partner

Having sex with a prostitute

Being a prostitute

Having sex with a virgin

Being a virgin or acting sexually inexperienced

Having sex with a priest, nun, or some other forbidden or inappropriate partner

Pretending to be a celebrity or fictional character

Having sex with a celebrity or fictional character

Trying out sexual approaches or positions that you may not actually be practicing in real life

Having sex while wearing the clothing of the opposite
sex, or being forced to do so
Having sex with a deity or a spiritual leader

Let your eyes roam over the list again, giving free rein to your imagination. Where there is imagination, there is creativity; where there is creativity, there is creation; where there is creation, there is sex. Flesh out each line with a picture in your mind, all the while knowing the source of the image, for therein lies the Way of Fantasy.

Zen Sex begins in the brain.

the way to zen sex

close your eyes and imagine your favorite sexual fantasy.

where does it come from?

where does it take you?

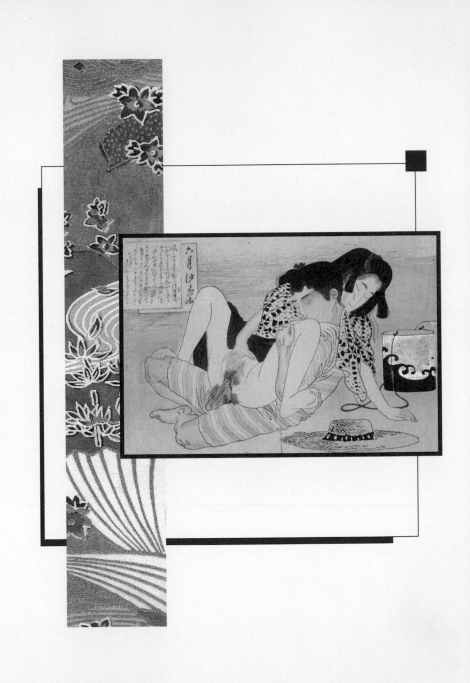

the way of discovery

The enjoyment of poetic beauty may well lead to hell.
But look what we find strewn all along our Path:
Plum blossoms and peach flowers!
—Ikkyu

As much as anything, Zen Sex is a process of discovery—self-discovery and the discovery of what your lover needs and desires. The more we know about ourselves, the more honest and open we can be with our lover. The more we know about our lover, the more satisfaction we can give. That's what makes for intimate, connected sex.

In *The Art of War*, a classic treatise on strategy written in 500 B.C., the Chinese general Sun Tzu says,

> *Know the enemy and know yourself; in a hundred battles you will never be in peril.*

> *When you are ignorant of the enemy but know yourself, your chances of winning or losing are equal.*

> *If ignorant of both your enemy and of yourself, you are certain in every battle to be in peril.*

We can look at Sun Tzu's words another way—as rules for anyone in a relationship. You don't have to view the world as a battle of the sexes; just substitute the word *partner* for *enemy*. Thus it follows:

> *If you know yourself and know your partner, your relationship will flourish.*

> *If you know yourself but don't know your partner, the road will be rocky.*

If you know neither yourself nor your partner, your relationship doesn't stand a chance.

All that matters in the Way of Discovery is our attitude in this moment—whether we're willing to engage in the process of discovery. To do so, we must keep an open mind and "carry an empty cup," as the zen masters say.

The empty-cup image stems from a famous parable about the visit of a university professor to the zen master Nan-in. The professor came to inquire about zen, but spent more time talking than listening.

Wordlessly, Nan-in began filling the professor's teacup until it overflowed onto the table.

"What are you doing?" the professor exclaimed.

"Like this teacup, you are full of your own opinions and theories," Nan-in replied. "How can I teach unless you first empty your cup?"

We are all like that professor at one time or another—unreceptive, focusing on our own needs when we should be paying attention to our lover's. Nan-in reminds us to catch ourselves in those moments and open our minds to discovery. The empty cup represents what zen masters call the "beginner's mind"—a mind that's newly born, open to learning, soaking up experience. That is the mind required for Zen Sex. After all, Zen Sex is not an end or a goal; it is a beginning. *Sex always leads to the Origin.* If you carry the beginner's mind to the bedroom, you are bound to discover something new.

It's said that in any given situation, one person is doing the teaching and one person is doing the learning. Let this rule apply inside the bedroom and out. You need not play out an overt teacher-student fantasy (although that might be fun); just be open to the cues and signals your lover sends you. Be of the mind to learn.

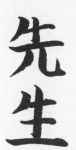

Sensei

The path of zen requires that we think of ourselves as both teacher and student at the same time—a concept implicit in the very word for teacher in Japanese: *sensei. Sensei* literally means "previous in life," or "one who has gone before." On the path of life, we look to those who have gone before us for guidance. For those coming after us on the path, we offer our life experience, what we know to be true. "When the student is ready, the teacher will appear," the zen masters say. See the two meanings here. When your mind is in a state of readiness to learn, you will learn; teachers will appear to you everywhere. Then, when you have learned enough, the teacher inside of *you* will appear, and you will guide others.

We all have something to learn from each other. Each of us has our own style and taste when it comes to lovemaking. On the path of Zen Sex, share yours, learn those of your partner, and discover new ones together.

A man once said, "What's sexy in bed is not the best-looking woman. What's sexy is what she wants to do to you, and what she wants done to her." Finding that out is the Way of Discovery. Don't expect your lover to know all your sweet spots. Frustration in a relationship often results when we expect our partner to be a mind reader and know what we want at any given moment. It's a common complaint: If our partners really loved us, they'd know what to do and what we want, without our having to tell them. Many a birthday and anniversary have been ruined because of that belief.

A lot of men and women want a technique that works every time on every lover. But what worked last time was last time; do not assume that the same moves will work this time, no matter how skilled in bed you may be. The moment is different; the mood is different. The Way of Discovery is to find out where your partner wants to go in *this* moment—how gentle, how firm, how fast, how slow. There are innumerable variations on the ways to love, awaiting your discovery in each moment. Finding your way is part of the fun of discovery. No need to get clinical or unsexy about it; on the contrary, your attitude of discovery should serve to heighten arousal. Let the sound of your partner's pleasure be your guide; those sighs and moans and cries carry the boundless mood.

Hearing them, you'll have no need to ask how your lover feels.

the way to zen sex

what part of your lover have you yet to explore?

find out tonight.

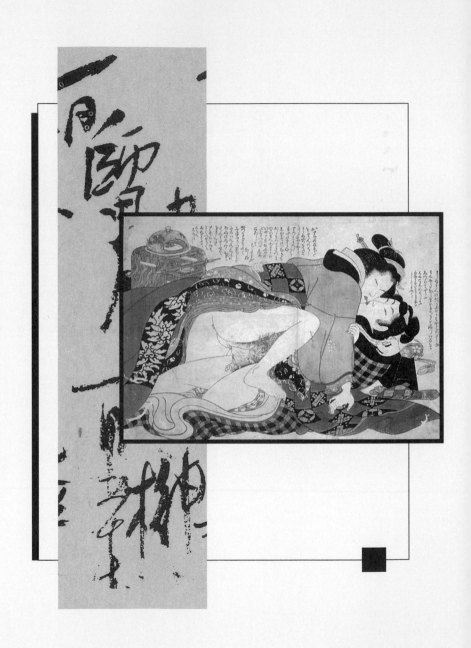

the way of initiating

White teeth smiling.
Brightness of skin.
On my seat in the high lama's row
At the quick edge of my glance
I caught her looking at me.
—Tsangyang Gyatso (1683–1706), sixth Dalai Lama

Sex, like life, takes action and participation. Someone has to make the first move.

You be the one.

Whenever we come to a crossroads, not knowing the next step to take; when we don't have a lover or our sex life is stuck in a rut—those are the moments we need to reach inside and initiate

positive action toward others. When in doubt, initiate. Say *yes*—
to love, to life, to joining in with others. That is how we stay on
the right path and, at the same time, elevate humanity.

The zen teacher Soen Nakagawa taught this lesson to a student who approached him during a meditation retreat. "I am
very discouraged," the student said. "What should I do?"

Soen's reply: "Encourage others."

We can always find a reason *not* to do something—we're too
tired; there's not enough time; it's the other person's turn. Reject
those reasons. The Way of Making Love lies in the doing.

If you find your sex life to be the same old same-old: Be of the
mind to break up your pattern. If your partner is always the
one to initiate, take the lead once in a while. You need not
equal the number of times your partner initiates the action;
maybe one time in ten will do the balancing.

Don't take the lead feeling that you have to; making love out
of a sense of duty is most unsexy. Do it because you want to.
Surprise your lover at a most unexpected time, in a most unexpected way, and you'll have a moment to remember for years to
come.

*If you're the one who always initiates and are tired of having to
do so:* Dig deeper and find new avenues of intimacy. Return to

the rituals of courtship; take a more romantic approach to wooing your partner; change the way you initiate. Inspired by your own creativity, you will not tire.

If your partner's sex drive is not compatible with your own: Talk to each other. A healthy relationship, even the most sexually compatible one, requires an ongoing process of negotiation. Both partners have to communicate their needs to each other, and look for ways to accommodate each other's needs on a day-to-day, moment-by-moment basis.

If two people truly attune to each other and care for one another, their disparate sex drives will naturally find a point of balance. They know that in the context of the larger relationship, sex is only one part. When an imbalance arises in the sexual area of their relationship, they balance it out in other areas—spending more nonsexual time together, perhaps, or giving each other more time to pursue their own individual interests. Those things, in turn, can help restore sexual harmony.

When two people fail to communicate their needs, or ignore those of their partner, the relationship is doomed to failure.

If you don't have a sex partner and would like one in your life: Take the initiative. But don't initiate out of neediness, or succumb to fear of rejection. Many women become accustomed to the man always initiating and hence never learn to risk making a first move. But if you follow the path of Zen Sex, you will know yourself and your worth. Let self-respect and love for life be the source of your actions. Then, should you encounter someone on your path who says *no*, your spirits will not sag.

That doesn't mean you proposition every person on the street. Just participate in the game of life: Open your eyes, open your arms to the world around you. The inward journey means nothing unless it opens you up to others. Be keen to the signals other people give you; you can miss them if you're not looking. Some people can't even tell when someone's flirting with them. They walk with their heads down, gazing at their feet, or enter a room trying to disappear into the walls. They need to carry an empty cup. That sense of *possibility* is what makes life exciting.

When the time comes to initiate, do not be afraid. That is the lesson of the zen nun Eshun, who studied as the lone woman among twenty monks. According to legend, one of the monks wrote Eshun a love letter, seeking to steal away with her in private.

The next day, Eshun and the monks gathered for a lecture. When the speaker finished, Eshun stood before the assembly and addressed the monk who had written her.

"If you really love me," she said, "come and embrace me now."

In the context of today's gender relations, we might think Eshun was trying to embarrass the letter writer in front of his peers. But the zen lesson of her action goes deeper than that. It speaks to acknowledging our true nature and embracing the moment as well.

If you love, Eshun says, love openly. The Way of Initiating is to become one with the source of love and let that love flow outward through you toward others. If your heart is pure, there is nothing to be ashamed of.

So many social forces turn people against their own hearts, making them close off. We tell people they can't love outside their race, their faith, their ethnic group. We tell gay people their love is immoral. The world is filled with Montagues and Capulets, obstructing love through pettiness and hatred. When people deny the love inside themselves or hide its expression, when they can't initiate love toward one another with open hearts, they damage their souls, and by extension, the soul of humanity.

A few words for those people already comfortable with initiating:

Be willing to initiate action, but don't overpursue a sexual relationship. You can go more than halfway to meet someone, but always leave room for him or her to come toward you. Show interest, but don't apply pressure.

If you find yourself pursuing someone and he blocks you or does not make a move to meet you, turn your attention elsewhere. To continue pursuit strays off the path into obsession.

If a person comes to meet you and then retreats, do not run after her. Wait at the line, but do not cross it. Allow time for confusion to settle. After a while, you can check to see if she wishes to meet you again. But proceed more slowly.

Understand the balance between yes and no. When someone says yes and then says no, respect the no, respect the person, and respect yourself.

When both parties say yes, let the fun begin.

the way to zen sex

make the first move tonight.

what will it be toward?

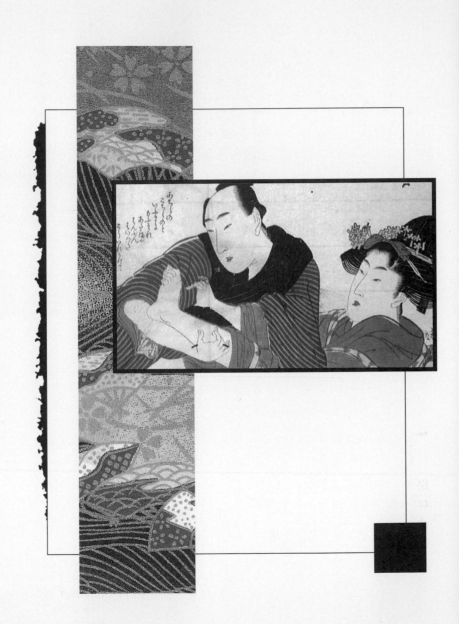

the way of anticipation

Day and night I cannot keep you out of my thoughts;
In the darkness, on an empty bed, the longing deepens.
I dream of us joining hands, exchanging words of love.
—Ikkyu

The next best thing to having sex is looking forward to sex. The Way of Anticipation is to revel in the tension of a good sexual buildup. Feel the edge of the moment, but stay relaxed. "My longing for you keeps me in this moment," said the mystical Sufi poet Rumi (1207–1273). Take a deep, long breath, and enjoy the feeling.

Whenever you feel as though you can't wait to have sex—wait. Let the moment come without rushing into it. We can all benefit from slowing down inside, whatever the action or occasion. When we rush, we lose the feeling of self-control. When we relax, we regain it. With control comes a feeling of confidence, and confidence is sexy.

Those who get too caught up in "doing it" inevitably short-change the preliminaries. They're thinking too much about what they *want* to be doing, instead of what they *are* doing. They fail to see the fun in getting there.

A zen parable about a young swordsman warns of this kind of overeagerness. The swordsman, Matajuro Yagyu, had been sent by his father to study with the master Banzo.

> *"If I work hard, how many years will it take me to become a master?" Matajuro asked.*
>
> *"Ten years," Banzo said.*
>
> *"If I work far more intensively," the student said, "how long would it take me?"*
>
> *Banzo estimated thirty years.*
>
> *"Why is that?" Matajuro said. "First you say ten and now thirty years. I will undergo any hardship to master this art in the shortest time."*

"Well," said Banzo, "in that case you will have to
remain with me for seventy years. A man in such a hurry
as you are to get results seldom learns quickly."

Banzo's lesson applies in the bedroom as well. Many young people, for example, are so eager to lose their virginity that they rush into sex long before they're ready. Even many mature adults make the mistake of sleeping together too soon, before they're emotionally prepared for a sexual relationship. In so doing, they fall into a relationship with the wrong person, or ruin the chance for a more lasting romance by getting too serious too fast. "Conquer haste," the zen masters say. The writer Joe Hyams, author of *Zen in the Martial Arts*, describes how he learned that lesson in a meeting with the master Bong Soo Han. The two were having tea when a letter arrived from the teacher's family in Korea. Hyams says,

Knowing he had been eagerly anticipating the letter, I
paused in our conversation, expecting him to tear open
the envelope and hastily scan the contents. Instead, he
put the letter aside, turned to me, and continued our
conversation.

The following day I remarked on his self-control,
saying that I would have read the letter at once.

"I did what I would have done had I been alone," he said. "I put the letter aside until I had conquered haste. Then when I set my hand to it, I opened it as though it were something precious."

I puzzled over this comment a moment, knowing he meant it to be a lesson for me. Finally I said I didn't understand what such patience led to.

"It leads to this," he said. "Those who are patient in the trivial things in life and control themselves will one day have the same mastery in great and important things."

The Way of Anticipation is to feel the edge of the moment and yet stay patient. In that period of sexual excitement right before you make love, conquer your haste; then set a hand to your lover like you're touching something precious. Looking too far beyond the moment is what leads to performance anxiety.

Even as you're making love, in the buildup toward climax, there should be a measure of relaxation. Says the sixth Dalai Lama, Tsangyang Gyatso,

The earth's spring essence wells up.
Since I met my lover
Body and mind have become relaxed.

The Way of Anticipation is to remain at ease, even as the heart races.

A relaxed spirit plays with the tension that precedes the point of orgasm, backing off and building up again and again according to the mood. Lose yourself in dalliance, absorbed in the moment. In lovemaking, there is no need to hurry toward a conclusion. Says Ikkyu,

> Amazing how many hours we spend in "sleep" [making love].
> Like butterflies we play endlessly.
> Hark! the bell chimes. Is it noon? or midnight?

When all awareness of time is lost, when we don't know whether it's noon or midnight, there can be no sense of rushing. Which is not to suggest that the buildup to every lovemaking session need be long and drawn out. In the balance of a good sexual relationship, the "quickie" can serve as a good change of pace. But even there, know the difference between quickness and rushing. The feeling of rushing is one of being pressed for time. When we feel pressed for time, we're not fully present in attending to our lover; our mind is elsewhere, watching the clock, running over the "to do" list. A good quickie is done not with a feeling of rushing, but *in the moment*.

When it's over, let the feeling linger, even as you button up your clothes and rejoin the party. Carry the Way of Anticipation into afterplay—those postcoital moments of intimacy and caress—for those are the moments that deepen the experience you and your lover have just been through.

Start looking forward to when you can do it again.

the way to zen sex

in that moment before the clothes come off tonight,
linger just a little bit longer.

tease your lover.

how does it make you feel?

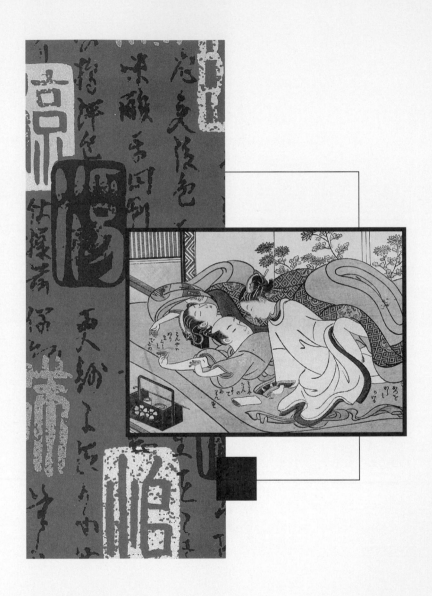

the way of surprise

Enlightenment comes by sudden experience.
Hui-neng (638–713)

Whether it's planting a sexy Polaroid in your lover's coat pocket or leaving an erotic message on the answering machine, there are two sides to the Way of Surprise: The giving of the surprise and the receiving of the surprise.

To surprise someone takes forethought—thinking in the moment about the moment to come. To be surprised is to get caught unawares. For each side, there is a decisive moment, and in that moment lies an opportunity for awakening.

Zen literature is replete with stories of the masters springing surprises, trying to elevate the awareness of their students. One story tells of Tokusan (781–867), during his early days of study with the teacher Ryutan. After a late night, Ryutan said, "The night is getting old. Why don't you retire?"

As Tokusan bowed and opened the door to leave, he said, "It is very dark outside."

Ryutan offered Tokusan a lighted candle. The instant Tokusan received it, the teacher blew it out.

In that moment of surprise, Tokusan's mind opened.

This is a key point in the Way of Surprise: *The surprise is for the benefit of the one being surprised.* Often we plan surprises for our own amusement, to see the startled look of a lover in a moment of embarrassment. But the true Way of Surprise is to give all thought to one's lover—to know what he wants or what she'd enjoy, and provide it out of love. In doing so, we elevate our own spirit and heighten our arousal. We recognize the routine in our lives and do something to break it up, thereby raising our awareness of love.

Anytime we're on the receiving end of a surprise is a chance to examine our reaction—to learn where our heart and head are. There will always be things that catch us off guard in life, intentional or otherwise. How we respond when there's no warning and no preparation offers a glimpse of who we really are.

A famous zen story illustrates the point. It involves an old woman in China who had supported a monk for more than twenty years. Such monks often received free lodging and food from townspeople in the belief that, if just one monk became enlightened, all of humanity would benefit.

The woman in this case began to wonder about the monk's progress. To find out, she enlisted the help of a girl who was "rich in desire."

"Go and embrace him," she told her, "and then ask suddenly: 'What now?'"

The girl called upon the monk and without much ado caressed him, asking him what he was going to do about it.

"An old tree grows on a cold rock in winter," replied the monk somewhat poetically. "Nowhere is there any warmth."

The girl returned and related what he had said.

"To think I fed that fellow for twenty years!" exclaimed the woman in anger. "He showed no consideration for your need, no disposition to explain your condition. He need not have responded to passion, but at least he should have evidenced some compassion."

She at once went to the hut of the monk and burned it down.

The surprise had revealed the monk's true nature. Twenty years of meditation had failed to produce a compassionate heart—the one true measure of progress in training. In the decisive moment, when there was no time to think, he had failed his test.

In a commentary on this story, the Indian guru Osho said the monk faced three possibilities. "One: If for twenty years he had not touched a beautiful woman, the first possibility was that he would be tempted, would be a victim, would forget all about meditation and would make love with this girl. The second possibility was that he would remain cold, controlled, and would not show any compassion towards this girl. He would simply hold himself back, hard, so that he could not be tempted. And the third possibility was: If meditation had come to fruition, he would be full of love, understanding, compassion, and he would try to understand this girl and would try to help her. She was just a test for these possibilities.

"If the first was the possibility, then all his meditation was simply a wastage. If the second was the possibility, then he had fulfilled the ordinary criterion of being a monk but he had not fulfilled the real criterion of being a man of meditation. . . . A man of compassion always thinks about you, about your need. He remained coldly self-centered. He simply said something about himself—'An old tree grows on a cold rock in winter—

nowhere is there any warmth.' He did not utter a single word about the woman. He did not even ask: 'Why did you come? Why? What do you need? And why have you chosen me out of so many people? Sit down.'. . . Love always thinks of the other; ego thinks only of oneself. Love is always considerate; ego is absolutely inconsiderate. Ego has only one language and that is of self. Ego always uses the other; love is ready to be used, love is ready to serve."

In his own commentary on the monk's story, Ikkyu says his reaction to the surprise would have been decidedly less cold:

> *The old woman was bighearted enough*
> *To elevate the pure monk with a girl to wed.*
> *Tonight if a beauty were to embrace me*
> *My withered old willow branch would sprout a new*
>   *shoot!*

As the saying goes, life is full of surprises. Let those remind you that you're alive—and full of love.

the way to zen sex

do something unexpected for your lover tonight.

surprise yourself by what you're willing to do.

z
s   e   x
n

surprise   63

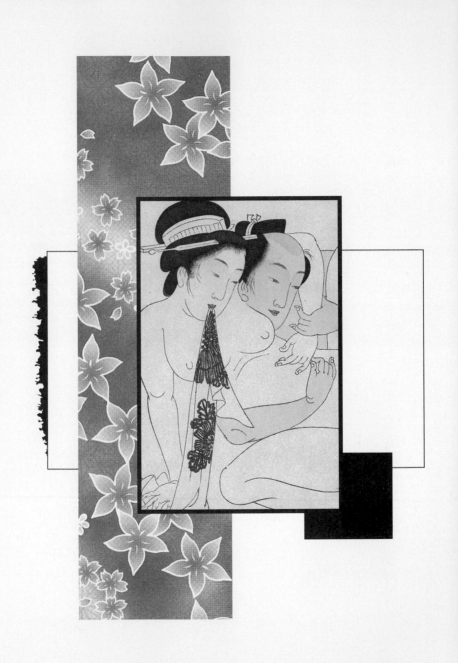

the way of the familiar

Though familiar with the soft flesh
Of my lover's body,
I cannot measure her depths.
—Tsangyang Gyatso, sixth Dalai Lama

They say familiarity breeds contempt. The Way of the Familiar breeds love.

If those electric first moments of a love affair start to fade with time, return to the beginner's mind of zen. In the bedroom, the path of familiarity remains ever tied to the path of discovery.

None of us starts out knowing our lover's style in bed, or even our own style. Through the Way of Discovery, we learn how to touch and give pleasure, try various ideas, experiment and explore. After a while, we come to know every pore of our partner's body, the texture and taste of the skin, the smell of the hair, the curves of the shoulders, the pleasure points unique to that one person. We know the other's fantasies and desires—and how to fulfill them.

Some lovers come to know so much that, after a while, they start to feel like they've done it all. Their sex lives fall into a rut; their lovemaking becomes routinized.

The Way of the Familiar is to reach that point and ascend to new heights.

There is a level of lovemaking that two people can get to only after sharing a lot of time together—time that can't be shortened or compressed, time that can only be lived. It is the same level reached by musicians who've played together for many years and come to know each other's thinking. No matter how talented they are individually, no group of musicians can sound like a real band if they haven't put in the time together playing.

In the Way of the Familiar, each lover has devoted time to training the other. When you know exactly how your lover likes it and your lover knows exactly how you like it, the lovemaking that ensues is guaranteed to be good.

That does not mean that every lovemaking session is the same and unvaried. To use the musical analogy again, a group that's played together for a long time may have a distinct sound, but it also has a vast repertoire of songs. Not every song gets played every night; the list changes according to the mood of the moment. And the best songs never grow old. No matter how many times they get played, they continue to offer fresh rewards. That is the feeling Tsangyang Gyatso describes when he says, "Though familiar with the soft flesh / of my lover's body, / I cannot measure her depths."

The Way of the Familiar is to continually explore those depths. Even if your lovemaking style is always the same, there are countless ways to make the familiar seem new. Make love in a new place. Make love in a new outfit. Make love to a new piece of music. Make love at a new time of day.

Each moment *is* new. *We have never lived it before and will never live it again.* It is familiar and unfamiliar at the same time.

We carry that feeling of "familiar unfamiliarity" forward by keeping our beginner's mind. The Buddha says as much in a parable about a man fleeing a tiger.

In the Buddha's story, the man runs from the tiger until he reaches a precipice. Swinging himself over the edge with a vine, the man looks down and sees another tiger below him. Suddenly, two mice, one white and one black, start to gnaw away at the vine.

Clinging for his life, the man sees a luscious strawberry growing near him. He plucks it and puts it in his mouth.

"How sweet it tasted!" the Buddha says.

How many strawberries had that man eaten in his life? After a time, they had become so familiar he had lost awareness of their inherent sweetness. The Buddha's lesson is to see the luscious strawberry and savor its sweetness in every moment.

We can get so accustomed to the beauty in our midst that we take it for granted. We ignore the reality that time is chasing us like a tiger. In this very moment, death is a single accident away. *Issun saki wa yami no yo*, the Japanese say: "One inch ahead and the world is pitch darkness." The Buddha implores us to treat every moment the same way—as though we were hanging over the edge of a cliff—and grab for that strawberry. Live like that and you will savor the taste of your lover. As the zen saying goes,

Each time you see it,
each time it's new

The saying stems from a core principle of the Japanese tea ceremony called *ichigo ichie*. Literally, *ichigo ichie* means "one time, one meeting."

Those who practice the Japanese tea ceremony, or *chado* ("the Way of Tea"), view it as a model for all human relations, romantic or otherwise. Each tea gathering is a unique moment in time, never to be repeated again. Even if the same people gather again the next day and repeat the same tea ceremony, they would occupy a different moment in time. In zen, there is only now. The past is past, the future an illusion. Only this moment offers the chance for enlightenment.

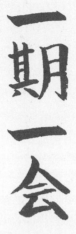

Ichigo ichie

The spirit of *ichigo ichie* is to experience this night of lovemaking, in this moment, to its fullest extent. No matter how familiar we are with each other, with our surroundings, we cannot get bored if we truly pay attention. Give thanks for the comfort of your lover sleeping next to you. Pay attention to the moment, the tea masters say, because it won't last forever.

None of us knows how long we have on this earth. And yet so many of us live as though we have time in abundance. We get lulled into complacency, mistaking the familiar for permanency. We think nothing ever changes. And yet, zen says,

sitting motionless, nothing happening—
spring coming, grass growing

See beneath the surface of things; feel the energy that makes the grass grow under our feet. It is the same energy we express through sex, through our very being. How can familiarity with this energy possibly breed contempt? We should long for such intimate familiarity.

When we live with the idea of *ichigo ichie*, we live in the spirit of that energy, loving life and love, making the most of every session of lovemaking. Familiar as our lover may be to us, we treat each night in the bedroom as special. We do not wait for a diagnosis of cancer to start savoring our lover's kiss. We do it now. Should tomorrow come, we do it again.

Living with the attitude of "one time, one meeting," we never have to ask, "Where did the time go?" We know.

It went to making love.

the way to zen sex

how many times have you made love to your lover?

remember your favorite details.

then make love again,

anew.

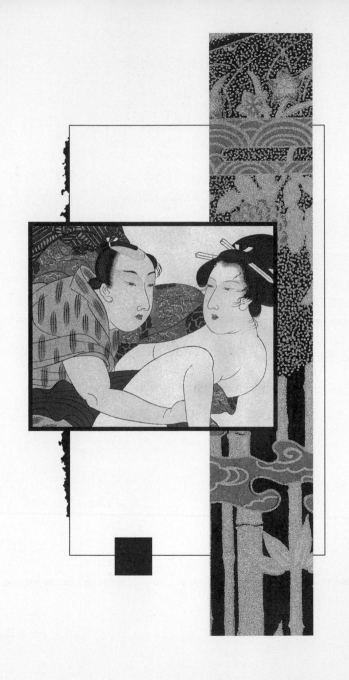

the seven ways of the body

The original body
Must return to
Its original place.
　　　—Ikkyu

the ways of Entering
　　　　　Accepting
　　　　　Touch
　　　　　Scent
　　　　　The Eyes
　　　　　The Mouth
　　　　　The Cry

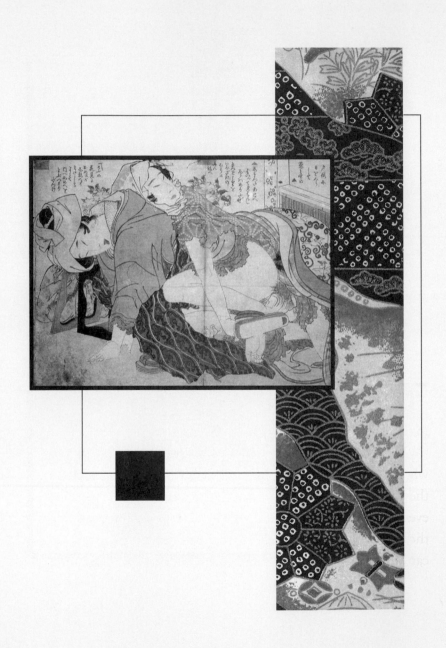

the way of entering

whispering all night even at sixty
I'm hard in her again and again.
—Ikkyu

The Way of Entering is known through the zen saying—
"Enter by form, exit from form." This has meaning on many levels.

On one level, the saying describes the path of artistry. It says, whenever you undertake something new—painting, cooking, the bedroom arts—first learn the basics. You don't need to know everything at once. Start out with small steps and proceed from there. Once you've internalized the rules of an art form, you can "exit from form" and create your own, personal expression.

In the bedroom, most people enter the world of sexual experience through masturbation. Before we engage in sex with a partner, we engage in sex with ourselves. Self-play introduces us to the pleasures of orgasm and how our sexual parts function; it prepares us for the more complex world of lovemaking. A virgin who masturbates may experience hundreds of orgasms before having sex with a partner, and may thus be more sexually at ease than someone who has never masturbated. To Ikkyu, masturbation offered the same opportunity for revelation as sex itself:

> *Eight inches strong, it is my favorite thing;*
> *If I'm alone at night, I embrace it fully—*
> *A beautiful woman hasn't touched it for ages.*
> *Within my* fundoshi *[underwear] there is an entire*
> *universe.*

From masturbation, we start learning how to make love. The idea becomes to "enter by form" physically, as one partner enters the other, and then "exit from form" spiritually, through transcendent sex.

To develop a level of artistry in bed, we may turn to sex manuals and videotapes, following the form of others, experimenting with different positions and techniques. But the ultimate aim is to transcend techniques; to get so good at them that we move beyond form and pattern and simply do what's natural. Forget all the information, Ikkyu says, and focus on the essence:

> *Every day, priests minutely examine the Dharma [zen teachings]*
> *And endlessly chant complicated sutras [sayings].*
> *Before doing that, though, they should learn*
> *How to read the love letters sent by the wind and rain, the snow and moon.*

Or, more bluntly, he says,

> *don't hesitate get laid that's wisdom*
> *sitting around chanting what crap*

The body has a wisdom all its own. Through the practice of forms, we develop that wisdom, in the same way that dancers and athletes develop muscle memory, until the day comes when we simply trust the body's wisdom without thinking. Thinking only gets in the way of the body's wisdom.

Each of us is born into a body at birth, and in the course of life we learn how to use and inhabit that body, discovering what gives it pleasure and the ways in which it melds with another. The Way of Entering reminds us that, at the most fundamental level, this is how we "enter by form": In the form of a human body. We "exit from form" when the body dies and our spirit is released—or through a transcendent realization, as in quiet meditation or in bed with a lover.

The zen nun Chiyono had such a realization one moonlit night while carrying a water pail bound with bamboo. When the bamboo broke and the bottom fell out of the pail, the nun had a flash of enlightenment. In the poem she wrote to commemorate the moment, the pail symbolized her physical body:

> In this way and that I tried to save the old pail
> Since the bamboo strip was weakening and about to
> break
> Until at last the bottom fell out.
> No more water in the pail!
> No more moon in the water!

Cling not to your body, Chiyono says. Empty yourself of ego and let your spirit flow out like water. Transcend this body that serves as your vessel; the opportunity is there to do so anytime, anywhere, in bed or out of bed.

Remember, too, that just as we enter the world *in* a body, we enter the world *through* a body as well—the body of our mother. The vagina that's entered in sex is the same opening through which life enters the world; the point of entrance is the point of exit, and the point of all beginning. Says Ikkyu,

> *It has the original mouth but remains wordless;*
> *It is surrounded by a magnificent mound of hair.*
> *Sentient beings can get completely lost in it.*
> *But it is also the birthplace of all the Buddhas of the ten*
>   *thousand worlds.*

Let the moment of penetration, when one lover physically enters the other, bring us back to our beginner's mind—and the origins of our body. Take care not to get lost. Through the Way of Entering, proceed straight in to the Source.

the way to zen sex

what form will your lovemaking take tonight?

how will you enter?

how will you exit?

z

s ⟳ x

n

entering 81

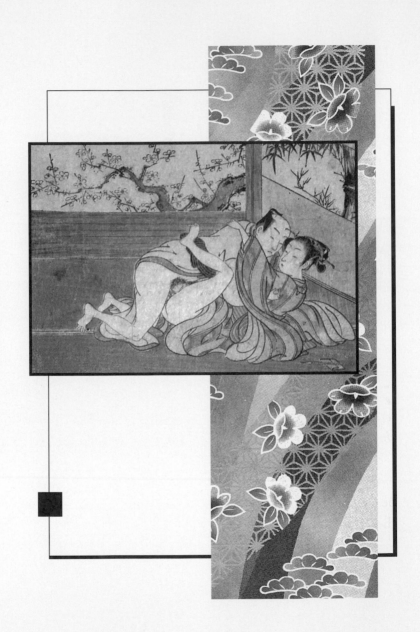

the way of accepting

don't worry please please how many times do I have to say it
there's no way not to be who you are and where
—Ikkyu

A popular recitation among people working through addictions is the "Serenity Prayer": *God, grant me the serenity to accept the things I cannot change, the courage to change the things I can, and the wisdom to know the difference.*

There is much zen in this.

The Way of Accepting is to accept those things that cannot be changed—not with resignation, but with joy. Chief among those things are:

Life
Ourselves
Our bodies
Our partner's body
What becomes of those bodies

Through diet, exercise, and surgery we can change the outward appearance of our bodies, but we cannot change the fact that, for as long as we live, we will inhabit those bodies, and that they will age. The Way of Accepting is to live with those facts, to be able to look in the mirror at any age and see oneself with smiling eyes.

The zen master Hotei once taught this Way of Accepting without uttering a single word.

Known for carrying a linen sack, Hotei was asked, "What is the significance of zen?" He plopped down his sack in silent reply.

The questioner continued, "Then, what is the actualization of zen?"

Hotei swung the sack over his shoulder and continued on his way.

Through the elegance of zen action, Hotei's first answer says, What is, is. Accept it. You plop down a sack. First the sack was over your shoulder, now it's down on the ground. Time moves on. That moment can never be repeated. The earth turns on its axis and revolves around the sun. Every minute we grow older. Somewhere someone is making love; somewhere else, someone is fighting a war. Someone is being born; someone is dying. All of those things are manifestations of the divine force that energizes the universe. That is the truth that underlies every action and every thing.

Hotei's second answer tells us how to live within that truth. Pick up your sack and go about your business. Participate in everyday life.

A lot of people mistake the attitude of acceptance for one of fatalism: "What will be, will be; there's nothing I can do about it." That is the mind of stagnation. Life is dynamic and changing, so to fully engage in life, we, too, must be dynamic and changing. The Way of Accepting is to take life as it comes— but *take* it. Like Hotei, pick up your sack and move on. What could be more ordinary? On the path of zen, such acceptance represents a miracle—the miracle of being alive.

As we learn to accept life as it comes, so do we learn the meaning of two of zen's central concepts: Imperfection and impermanence.

Imperfection

In zen thinking, life is perfectly imperfect. Like sex, it's messy, complicated, exhilarating, confusing—and ultimately a miracle. With all its hassles, that is how life is meant to be. Even as we realize the imperfection of human beings, we understand that, on a divine level, everything is perfect just the way it is.

Through Zen Sex, we bring the same attitude to our relationships. People are who they are. We can encourage them to change their behavior, but in the end, only they can change themselves. It's we who must look to make a change within ourselves and learn to live with the other's "imperfections."

Our media feed us so many images of beautiful people living beautiful lives that our own lives can seem inadequate by comparison. Against all logic, we measure ourselves and our loved ones against an impossible standard. But the Japanese have a saying, *Meiba ni kuse ari*: "Even the famous horse smells." You can fantasize about how much better life would be if you could marry a movie star or sleep with a supermodel, but your dream denies the reality: Even the famous wake up with bad breath in the morning and have their problems in bed.

The zen mind knows how to see the beauty in life's imperfection. If all things speak of the divine, then all things have an inherent beauty. Whether or not we can see it depends on our level of awareness. If we can attune ourselves through zen, we come to understand what the masters mean when they say,

"Beauty can be coaxed out of ugliness." Penetrate to the essence of a thing and you will see the radiance at its source.

Once we learn to see that inner radiance, much of our unhappiness evaporates. We get past the hang-ups with our appearance or our partner's; instead of seeing flaws, we feel good in our skin. We recognize our body as merely a vehicle of the spirit, and understand that for all the imperfections of the outward package, the source of that package is perfect and divine. We identify not with the surface of the being, but with the sexual energy at its core.

In this way do two imperfect lovers make perfect love.

Impermanence
Inevitably the body will die. But so long as you inhabit one, live with joy. The Way of Accepting is not to accept death, but to accept *life*.

In a single act of lovemaking, we can transcend the limits of the physical body and realize the divine reality within the present moment. What could make a person feel more alive?

Our natural impulse is to fear the threat of death to our bodies. Zen masters call that fear "clinging to dust"—the material dust of life. Nothing in this material world will go with you in death, not your body, your money, or your possessions.

Everything moves from ashes to ashes and dust to dust; we must learn to accept that, and, through zen, to penetrate to the deeper truth of our existence. In an essay called "Skeletons," Ikkyu writes,

> *We appear as skeletons covered with skin, male and female, and lust after each other. When the breath expires, though, the skin ruptures, sex disappears, and there is no more high or low. Underneath the skin of the person we fondle and caress right now is nothing more than a bare set of bones. Think about it—high and low, young and old, male and female, all the same. . . . This is how the world is. Those who have not grasped the world's impermanence are astonished and terrified by such change. . . . Free yourself from form and return to the original ground of being.*

We free ourselves from form through lovemaking, using the body to transcend its very impermanence. We come to see our essence not as the body that contains our sexual energy, but as the sexual energy itself, which is eternal. Our essence is like fire. Too often we mistakenly see ourselves as the candle.

In our hearts we know that a full expression of love, one that emanates from the source of life, carries on long after the body expires. When the zen master Ryokan expressed his love for the nun Teishin, he promised eternal love:

If your heart
Remains unchanged,
We will be bound as tightly
As an endless vine
For ages and ages.

Entwine with your lover like an endless vine. Accept each other in this moment and return to the original ground of your being.

Therein lies serenity.

Therein lies love.

the way to zen sex

make love with your partner in front of a mirror.

accept all you see,

and smile.

z
s e x
n

accepting 91

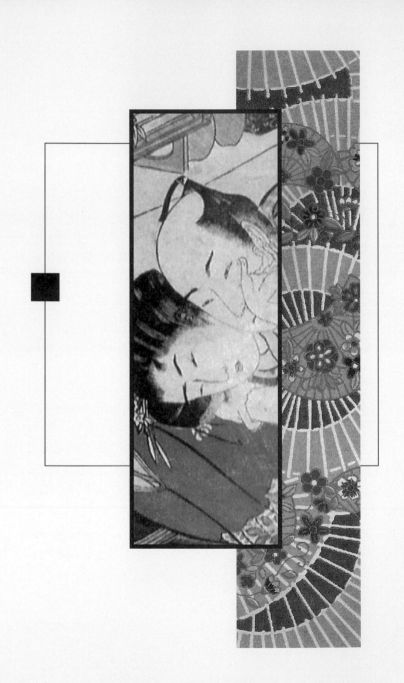

the way of touch

she'd play with it almost anywhere day and night
touch it with the deepest part of herself
—Ikkyu

From the moment we're born, we need the touch of another. In hospital incubators, premature babies are regularly stroked and massaged, lest they become psychologically and physically stunted. From the moment of birth, touch tells us that we're not alone in this world, that we're safe and loved. Throughout our lives, we never outgrow the need for that kind of touch. Sadly, some of us never get it, or stop getting it when we reach a certain age.

Touch communicates feelings on a deep, immediate level. Anger, tenderness, love, tension, support, desire—all of those things come across in the merest contact. Sexual touch, for the most part, is unmistakable. When certain zones of the body are touched in a certain way, no words need be spoken. The message is clear: *I want you.*

Sexual touch is also the most intimate. Relatively speaking, there are very few people we allow to touch us in that way, and very few who grant us the same privilege. The Way of Touch is to acknowledge that privilege and recognize how special it is.

There is nothing like the sensation of crossing the line into sex with another person for the first time, hands suddenly free to roam wherever they want, off to explore new skin and shape, feeling those points of softness and solidity. Many people become addicted to the excitement, so they change lovers in a constant search for newness.

As anyone who's been in an extended relationship knows, after a while, the sense of touch loses that special tingle. Just as we no longer feel a wristwatch after we've been wearing it for a while, we can become so accustomed to the feel of our lover that our senses take it for granted.

If we make ourselves aware of that wristwatch, though, we can feel it. Not only that, we can feel it with more depth, because we're focusing on it. The Way of Touch is to take the same approach to our lover. Whether new or familiar, concentrate on your lover's touch, just as you concentrate on touching your lover.

Often, the touching aspect of sex gets overlooked in the eagerness to move on to the main course. Take the time to touch each other before and after sex. In fact, no matter what the time of day, touch your lover whenever you're within reach. Lean a head on the shoulder, wrap an arm around the waist. Hold hands. Play footsie. Scratch your lover's back. Above all, touch with love and gratitude. Let your partner *feel* it. Touch is the *only* way we physically connect with one another.

The great love of Ikkyu's life was a blind musician known as Lady Mori. In numerous poems he rhapsodized about the skill of her hands, whether she was playing an instrument or caressing his body. Even Ikkyu, at the height of zen awareness, could not summon the depth of feeling and sensitivity she brought to her touch.

My hand is no match for that of Mori.
She is the unrivaled master of love play:
When my jade stalk wilts, she can make it sprout!
How we enjoy our intimate little circle.

It's so easy for the mind to drift off sometimes, to become disconnected from our touch. How quickly the tender strokes of a lover can turn impatient, groping, insensitive to the mood. The Way of Touch is like that of Lady Mori—loving and assured, playing her partner like an instrument, releasing the song inside.

Many people think that lovemaking is all a matter of technique—finding the right spots to rub and tickle. But just as in music, no amount of technique makes up for a lack of soul. The best sex, like the best music, is uplifting because we put our whole heart into it.

What a gift it is to be able to touch someone so intimately—the kind of touch that makes a person happy to be alive.

Make someone happy tonight.

the way to zen sex

close your eyes so as to sharpen your sense of touch.

imagine your lover's body as an instrument.

play your favorite love song.

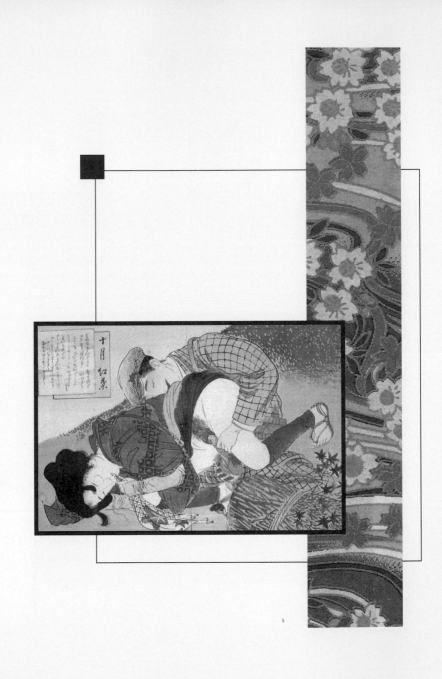

the way of scent

The perfume from her narcissus causes my bud to sprout,
sealing our love pact.
The delicate fragrance of the flower of eros,
A waterborne nymph, she engulfs me in love play,
Night after night, by the emerald sea, under the azure sky.
—Ikkyu

The Way of Scent is beyond words. It can be known only by living and breathing.

When certain smells pass through the nose, we know them instantly: The scent of a lover's clothes. The scent of a lover's hair. The scent of a lover's sex. Hours after the person is gone, the scent of a lover's pillow can comfort us through a lonely night.

Try to describe those smells to someone, though, and words fail. We can talk about a lover's features and our friends get a vivid mental picture—height, weight, hair color, eye color, build—and we can mimic the way a person sounds, but how can we describe a lover's scent? As "clean"? "Intoxicating"? We can get specific if we name the perfume or cologne, but even then, how can we specify what Chanel No. 5 smells like to someone who doesn't know?

The inadequacy of words in the realm of scent is perfectly suited for zen. Zen does not reject the use of words, but it clearly has limited use for them. "Words are the fog one has to see through," goes a zen saying. In fact, anyone who tries to define zen in words is considered a fool. As U.S. Supreme Court Justice Potter Stewart once said of obscenity, "I can't define it, but I know it when I see it." So it is with zen. Zen simply *is*. We call it "zen" to give it a name, but the name means nothing; it doesn't describe anything, because zen can't be known through words. The limits of words led Ikkyu to say,

> *It is easy to be glib about zen—I'll just keep my mouth*
> * shut*
> *And rely on love play all the day long.*

Like zen itself, the Way of Scent is to experience the world directly, without words. Zen awareness results from direct, immediate perception of the world, before our thoughts get tangled up in words.

This is why zen teaching relies so heavily on paradox. It deliberately uses words against words to wipe the mind clean of words and back to our immediate, wordless perception.

Once, the zen master Joshu (778–897) was working in the garden when a monk asked for a lesson in the essence of zen.

"Cypress tree in the garden," came the reply.

Joshu's answer sounds meaningless on the surface. But his words have been passed down through the generations as a clue to enlightenment. They sprang from his direct perception of the world without any intellectual mediation. To him, it was the only way to use words to describe the indescribable.

In commenting on Joshu's lesson, the zen master Mumon (1183–1260) says,

Words cannot describe everything.
The heart's message cannot be delivered in words.
If one receives words literally, he will be lost,
If he tries to explain with words, he will not attain
*   enlightenment in this life.*

Through the Way of Scent, we find that same place of word-lessness, using our sense of smell to experience the everyday indescribable. With each breath, each inhalation of air, comes a new opportunity for enlightenment. In the scent of his lover, Ikkyu found universal truth:

and the nights inside you rocking
smelling the odor of your thighs is everything

Breathe in your lover's essence, letting no words enter your mind. Then, when someone asks you to describe the smell, you can answer without thought, as Joshu did:

Lover in the bedroom.

the way to zen sex

turn out the lights.
turn down the sound.
breathe.

find the scent of your lover.

never forget that smell.

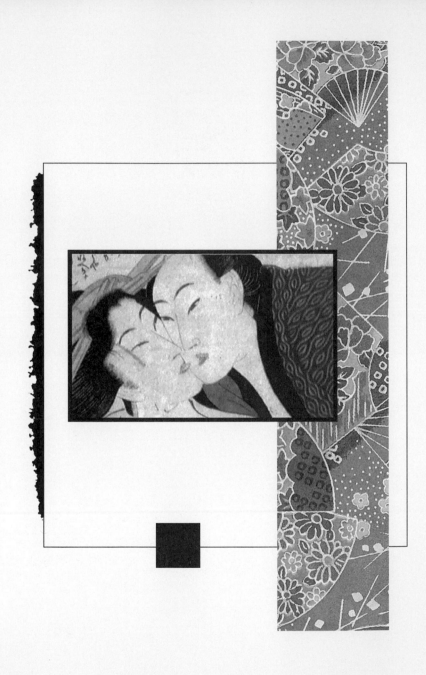

the way of the eyes

believe in the man facing you now
just narrow your eyes feel the deep love
—Ikkyu

The Way of the Eyes is known through what they see and
what they show.

What they see is light.

What they show is spirit.

Ultimately, the two are the same.

We tend to look at the world from a sense of separateness—
that there's someone "in here" looking at the world "out there."
In reality, we're always apart from, and *a part of,* the larger

world around us. To live in zen is to be aware of both positions at once.

Gazing out at the world, our eyes, at their most fundamental level, are simply light sensors—organs responding to electromagnetic radiation that stimulates our central nervous system. It's light that enables us to find our lover in a crowd, watch each other undress, or, as Ikkyu describes, take in the pleasurable sight of a companion:

> *at the bath she bathed scrubbing her face and body*
> *at the bath I splashed water on myself enjoying her body*

The eye is instinctively drawn to what it finds sexy. Throughout nature, from the brilliant orange fins of the guppy to the flashy plumage of the peacock to the jeans that fit just so on the human body, males and females of various species use visual cues to show off their sexuality. We respond to these on a purely animal level. Unconsciously, our pupils expand when we're sexually excited. Researchers found that men, when asked to rate the attractiveness of women in a set of photographs, were more attracted to those with dilated pupils, and that in response, the pupils of the men would dilate as much as 30 percent. It's as though when we see something sexy, the eye wants to let more of that gorgeous light in. As the troubadour poet Guiraut de Borneilh wrote,

> *The eyes are the scouts of the heart,*
> *And the eyes go reconnoitering*
> *For what it would please the heart to possess.*

Too often, though, we become preoccupied with surface appearances. The Way of the Eyes is to see through to the essence of things. Our pupils may dilate at a sexy visage, but as human beings, we also have the capacity to reflect on what we see. In many cases, our seeing is more "looking at" than true seeing, says Frederick Franck, author of *Zen Seeing, Zen Drawing*:

> *Merely* looking-at *the world around us is immensely different from seeing it. Any cat or crocodile can look-at things and beings, but only we humans have the capacity to see. Although many of us, under the ceaseless bombardment of photographic and electronic imagery that we experience daily, have lost that gift of seeing, we can learn it anew, and learn to retrieve again and again the act of seeing things for the first time, each time we look-at them.*

The failure to truly see one another leads directly to pain in sexual relations. "When a man looks at a woman and sees only somebody to go to bed with," says the mythology scholar Joseph Campbell, "he is seeing her in relation to a fulfillment of some need of his own and not as a woman at all. It's like looking at cows and thinking only of roast beef." At bottom, that failure is a blindness to the inherent divinity of all things. When we abuse nature or other human beings, we are failing to see the Light behind the light.

The Way of the Eyes is to see that great Light, the spiritual luminescence of all things. Make a meditation of what's before your eyes; absorb yourself in it. In the words of James Joyce, "Any object, intensely regarded, may be a gate of access to the incorruptible eon of the gods." *Stare at it until your eyes drop out,* Ikkyu says, *this desk this wall this unreal page.* Do so until you recognize *who* is staring—not "you" in your ego-shell, but the source of you. It is the same spirit as that of the Light. That's the true meaning of the adage, "The eyes are the mirror of the soul."

We, all of us, are the divine spirit gazing upon itself in a gigantic mirror. As Ikkyu says,

> *mirror facing a mirror*
> *nowhere else*

The simple act of reflection gives meaning to human existence. Thomas Berry, a scholar of world religions, says our reflection is the primary contribution of human beings to the universe:

> We enable the universe to reflect on itself and in a
> sense to smile at and enjoy itself. While the universe
> activates itself in each part of the universe, the special
> attribute of the human is to enable the universe to reflect
> on itself with a special mode of intelligible self-
> awareness, to enjoy itself and to celebrate itself in the
> light of the numinous mystery that is expressed in
> everything.

Now gaze into the eyes of your lover and see your own reflection. As your pupils dilate in their irises, the circles growing within circles, ask yourself:

Who is looking at whom?

the way to zen sex

exhaust your partner in passionate lovemaking.

as he drifts off to sleep, meditate on him with your eyes.

what does the light reveal?

z

s   🌀   x

n

the eyes   *111*

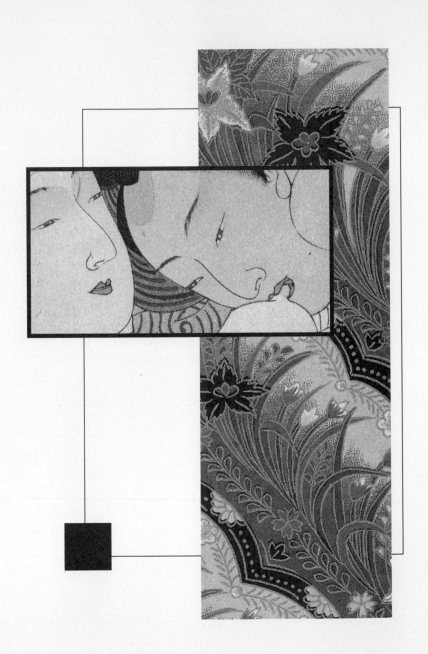

the way of the mouth

I am infatuated with the beautiful Mori from
the celestial garden.
Lying on the pillows, tongue on her flower stamen,
My mouth fills with the pure perfume of the waters
of her stream.
Twilight comes, then moonlight shadows,
as we sing fresh songs of love.
—Ikkyu

Through the mouth we consume that which gives us life.
We find sustenance in the outer world, swallow it, and it
becomes part of us.

The Way of the Mouth is to take the same approach in sex. Devour your lover. Use your mouth over every inch of your partner's body in every way that you can. Think of the all delicious things you can do with the lips, tongue, and teeth—then do them:

kiss
    lick
        nibble
           taste
              bite
                  suck
                    eat
                      blow
                        drink
                        swallow

On a Scrabble board, none of these words would cause anyone to blush. But in a sexual context, they arouse the mind and cause the pulse to race. Let this be a reminder that the mouth serves a verbal function in lovemaking, too. Those attuned to the Way of the Mouth know the aphrodisiac power of erotic talk. Whether whispered at a dinner party, spoken frankly over the phone, or screamed in mid-coitus, the words we put in a lover's ear can set the soul ablaze. Nasty, naughty, nice, all of the above—say what you want and what you want to do. The bedroom is no place for silence. Beg. Plead. Tease. *Command* your lover. The point is to peak your partner's—and your own—physical arousal. Just as zen uses words to escape the limits of words, so too should sex talk propel us toward that moment of transcendent release.

The mouth has a deeply erotic place in the human psyche. Anthropologists, for example, say that one reason men and women find the lips so seductive is their resemblance to the moist and swollen labia of sexual arousal. In mouth-to-mouth kissing, with its exchanging of fluids and insertion of tongues, we symbolically inflame the labia and return to our point of entry into the world.

We make a similar return through oral sex. To Ikkyu, life offered no greater delight than making love with the mouth. As a master of the Japanese *shakuhachi* flute—a demanding instrument on the lips and tongue—he relished transferring his mouth skills to a woman's genitalia. To him, cunnilingus could end a man's spiritual searching:

> *all koans just lead you on*
> *but not the delicious pussy of the young girls I go*
>   *down on*

He returned to the theme of oral sex again and again during his long romance with the musician Lady Mori:

> plum blossom close to the ground her dark place opens
> wet with the dew of her passion wet with the lust of my
>   tongue

> I'd sniff you like a dog and taste you
> then kiss your other mouth endlessly if I could white hair
>   or not

> once while she was cooking I kneeled put my head
>   between her warm dark legs
> up her skirt kissed and licked and sucked her until she
>   came

> I remember one quiet afternoon she fished out my cock
> bent over played with it in her mouth for at least an
>   hour

As Ikkyu's poetry notes, oral sex requires a higher level of skill than most aspects of lovemaking. It involves more technique, more sensitivity, more service, more practice. It's one area of the love arts where we can pursue the course of mastery if we so choose. As with the study of zen, we need no special talent to progress; all who want to learn the art, can. It simply comes down to one's hunger to do it.

Use your mouth every which way you can and consume your lover with hunger. Take nourishment in your partner. Fill your insides with your lover's essence, and savor the taste.

The Way of the Mouth can be the gateway to enlightenment.

the way to zen sex

kiss your lover's mouth throughout intercourse.
feel the circle created.

where does it begin?
where does it end?

z
s **e** x
n

the mouth   119

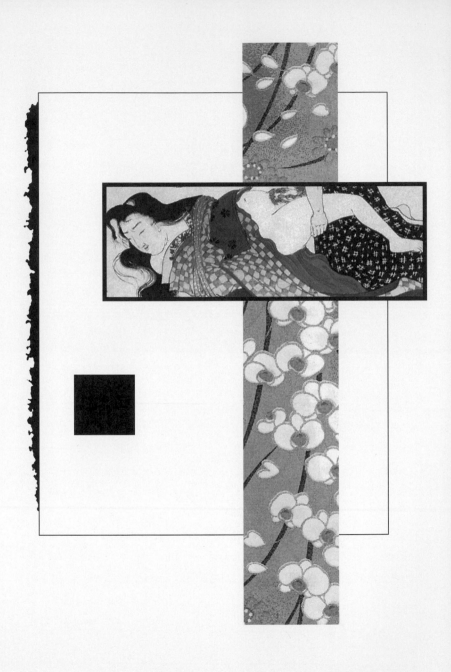

the way of the cry

*something in us always wants to cry out
someone we love knows hears*
—Ikkyu

In zen, every sound is the song of the divine spirit, an expression of the ultimate truth. When making love, this truth is known through the Way of the Cry.

A zen story tells of a master who had prepared a sermon for his students. As he opened his mouth to speak, a bird sang.

"The sermon has been delivered," the master said.

There, in the song of a bird, we can hear nature's truth. The same is true in the sounds of sex. The sighs, moans, and screams we express during lovemaking emanate from a place deep within—unselfconscious expressions of what we feel in the moment. Like the mating call of birds, they represent natural expressions of the sexual energy at our core. Enlightenment awaits anyone with ears attuned enough to hear it.

Zen masters put a special emphasis on hearing, most famously in the koan of Hakuin (1689–1769) asking students to ponder *sekishu no onjo*: "the sound of one hand clapping." When monks sit in long hours of meditation, they become absorbed in the sound of their own breathing and the sounds of nature—the chirp of a bird, the breeze in the trees, the buzz of an insect. They seek to penetrate the place of no sound and no silence—the *source* of sound and silence. The only man-made sound they hear is the toning of a bell, or the clack of wooden blocks, signaling the end of a meditation session, which heightens the sense of surrounding silence.

In zen, every sound and every silence carries equal weight. Ikkyu's breakthrough to enlightenment came through the cawing of a crow. But it was the silence between the caws that struck him. His master bestowed the name Ikkyu on him because it meant "one pause." As Ikkyu later wrote,

one pause between each crow's
reckless shriek Ikkyu Ikkyu Ikkyu

The notion of one pause between shrieks signifies the zen view of time as an endless chain of existence, with each lifetime but a brief interval. Through the Way of the Cry, we realize the same truth. Our time on this earth is short. To live it well, fill it with love. *Make love* in the fullest sense of those words. We must connect our one pause here to the great continuum of time. The sound of sexual excitement welling up from the ground of our being is the voice of the God-spirit within. Hearing it, expressing it, we feel the power of something greater than ourselves. The challenge of living in one pause is to hear that power in *every* sound, and in every silence as well.

Zen masters use a particular shout—*katsu!*—for just that effect. It is an expression of pure spirit, emanating from one's source, the same as the cry of love during sex. The zen master Rinzai was famous for his *katsu*, startling monks at the precise moment to awaken them to zen truth. Ikkyu, who idolized Rinzai, remarked in one poem,

> *Rinzai screamed KATSU! at precisely the right time gave*
> *life death KATSU!*
> *eyes everywhere blazing blazing eyes sun moon KATSU!*
> *KATSU!*

In the heat of passion, the cry of a lover can produce the same revelation. We hear it and become energized; we push our lover higher and higher in release, sending back the energy in an expanding circle.

When the cry of love escapes from you, let it sing from the deepest part of yourself. Says Ikkyu, "Ten thousand sutras [religious sayings] are distilled in a single song." All who hear the song will recognize the ecstatic truth, the release of a boundless energy too strong for the body to contain.

Call it the sound of pleasure.

Call it the sound of Sound.

Whatever you call it: Call out.

the way to zen sex

riding your naked lover tonight,

sing your mating song.

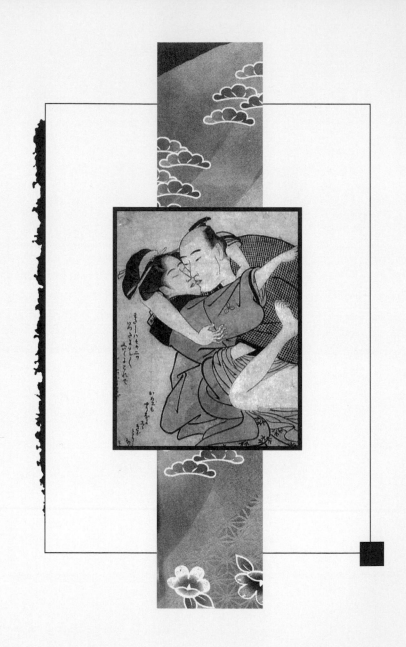

the seven ways of the spirit

*this hungry monk chanting by lamplight is Buddha
and he still thinks of you*

                              —Ikkyu

the ways of Interplay
        Giving
        Clouds
        Union
        Release
        Creation
        Birth and Rebirth

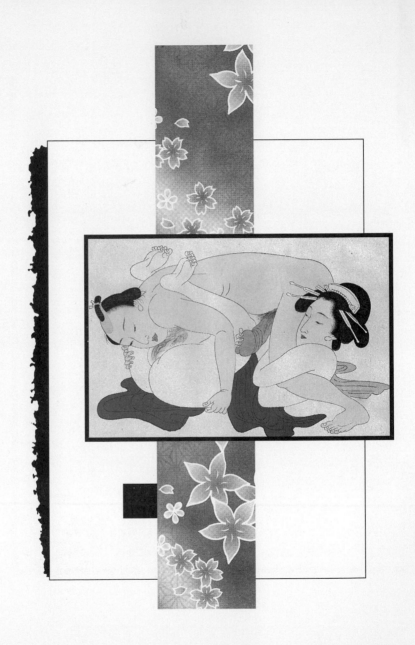

the way of interplay

*Night after night, we two lovebirds snuggle
on the meditation platform,
Lost in dalliance, intimate talk, and orgasmic bliss.*
—Ikkyu

The Way of Interplay is to understand the rhythmic give-and-take inherent in any relationship—the interplay of yin and yang.

Yin-yang is an ancient Chinese cosmology symbolized by interlocking fetal figures of black and
white. Together, yin and yang represent the
pairs of opposites that make up our experience
of the cosmos: male and female; life and death;

love and hate; matter and void. In Eastern thinking, these pairs of opposites go on endlessly, in infinite variety. Here are some of the characteristics commonly associated with yin and yang:

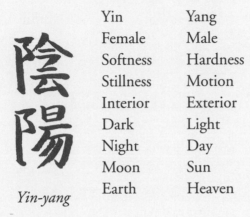

Yin	Yang
Female	Male
Softness	Hardness
Stillness	Motion
Interior	Exterior
Dark	Light
Night	Day
Moon	Sun
Earth	Heaven

Yin-yang

Like two partners whose lovemaking moves through changing positions, yin and yang are not static, but in constant ebb and flow—not separate but united; opposed and yet engaged. One does not exist without the other; the two make up a single whole. "Opposites and differences define and explain each other," says the *Tao Te Ching*, "and their shifting balance maintains the harmony of things."

Zen Sex requires an awareness of the interplay between these pairs of opposites, for collectively, they shape the way we experience the world and especially sex. In fact, sex may be the best way to understand the interplay of yin and yang. Nothing more clearly illustrates the idea of "the two that are one and the one that is two" than a pair of lovers entwined, both whole unto themselves and yet half of a larger whole.

To grasp the depth of this interplay, note that within the larger circle of yin and yang, each fetal figure contains a small circle of the other. That is to say, there are circles within circles within circles. Nothing and no one is completely yin or completely yang. All of us contain a male and female side; we are all born equally of one man and one woman. One side may seem to dominate the other, but remember, there is always a broader yin-yang balance to consider, just as there is always a smaller one.

If we insist, for example, that all relationships conform to the male-female model, we fail to see the whole picture of yin and yang. Every relationship has its own balancing of yin and yang, not only those that are male-female, but those that are male-male or female-female as well. (Historically, homosexuality did not carry the same stigma in Japanese temples as in the Western church, and was an accepted lifestyle for zen priests. Ikkyu indicates that his early sexual experiences were with young boys: "This beautiful . . . lad is like one branch of plum," he once wrote. "If you want to know this flower, be tender.")

A same-sex partnership might look like two yangs without a yin, but within the relationship, one partner may be more feminine (yin) and the other more masculine (yang). On a societal level, homosexuality can be seen as a smaller circle within the larger circle of the heterosexual world—or in some communities, the larger circle containing a smaller circle of heterosexuals.

The Way of Interplay is constantly in flux, like an ocean rising and receding. Because of that, we can never strike a perfect state of balance between yin and yang. Instead, we must engage in an active process of balanc*ing*, like lovers walking across the hull of a boat rocking at sea. Through this ongoing process, we follow the great Middle Way that transcends the pairs of opposites and leads to enlightenment.

The Way of Interplay is to harmonize yin and yang within and without—in ourselves, our sex lives, and the world around us. The back-and-forth nature of yin and yang gives it an underlying rhythm. The challenge is to feel that rhythm and move to it.

We often hear people say they have no natural rhythm, but what is their heartbeat if not a rhythm? Their pulse? The rhythm of yin-yang is at our core, in the inhale-exhale of our breath, in the left-right swing of our gait. If we go looking for our natural rhythm, we're out of sync with ourselves, because we're searching for something we already have.

In Japanese, the word for "natural rhythm" is *hyoshi*. Literally, it means "child's clap." We all have this innocent sense of rhythm inside; we're born with it. When we feel it, we can align our rhythm with the rhythm of yin-yang around us—the rhythm of our lover; the rhythm of the day and the season; the very rhythm of the cosmos. "The goal of life," says the mythology scholar Joseph Campbell, "is to make your heartbeat match the beat of the universe."

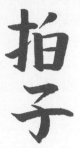

Hyoshi

The more we live in rhythm with yin-yang, the more we develop a sense of pace and timing. We learn to set our own pace and conform to no other. We learn how fast or slow to proceed in a relationship, when to escalate it or break it off. We learn how to build sexual tension—how long to kiss, how long to pet, how long to hold off the point of release. We learn when to lead and when to follow, for the Way of Interplay demands familiarity with both. As the zen masters say, *Ryusui saki o arasowazu*: "Flowing streams do not compete with one another." Flow together with your partner; make love naturally.

The rhythm of interplay is not something to think about. It can't be known through the mind. We have to *live* it, both aware and unaware of it at the same time. When the music is right, the clothing is shed, and the lighting falls just so across your lover's body, there is no thought to rhythm. Only when the phone suddenly rings or the wrong word is said in the midst of passionate lovemaking do we become consciously aware of the rhythm, because it has been broken.

Those attuned to the Way of Interplay realign their rhythm; those who aren't so attuned will find the moment and mood lost. The way to recapture a broken rhythm is to enlarge your sense of rhythm. When the flow toward climax is interrupted, expand your concept of what constitutes a single lovemaking session. Consider, for example, the thinking of the master samurai engaged in a duel. A lesser swordsman might attack, get blocked, and find his rhythm disrupted by his opponent. But the skilled samurai maintains his rhythm through a whole series of parries, because each strike and thrust is not a separate move but *incorporated into one continuous movement* toward the objective of victory. Use that kind of thinking to enlarge your sense of rhythm in the bedroom. Don't let an interruption in lovemaking break the mood for good. If you're frolicking in bed on a weekend afternoon and there's an insistent knock on the door, keep the feeling of moving toward consummation—even if you can't resume until hours later. Use your eyes, your voice, your hands, your toes in those intervening hours to remind your lover of what awaits the moment the guests go home.

When you resume, feel the rhythm of yin and yang between yourselves and grow your circle as one.

follow your lover's lead, leading your lover along.
play with each other.
move in and out together,
two into one,
sometimes faster,
sometimes slower,
sometimes deeper,
sometimes harder

who are the two?
what is the one?

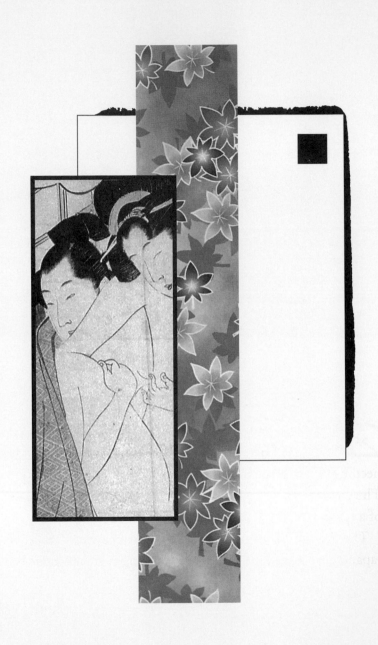

the way of giving

Ikkyu still sings aloud each night to himself
  to the sky the clouds
    because she gave herself freely
    her hands her mouth her breasts her long moist thighs
      —Ikkyu

Zen Sex is simply this: Lovers making love, giving to the other, *wanting* to give to the other—not taking, not needing, not selfish, but selfless and devoted in this moment. The challenge is to carry that spirit through to every moment of a relationship.

The Way of Giving is based on the teachings of *chado,* the Japanese tea ceremony. Each tea gathering is a chance for host and guest to commune together in the singleness of the moment. The host shows the guest every consideration; the guest reciprocates with gratitude. In this small way, the two create harmony between themselves, and thus, in the broader world.

One of the fundamental principles of *chado* applies directly to giving. It is called *kokoro ire*, or "inclusion of the heart's spirit." Just put your heart into what you do, the tea masters say. Don't serve tea out of a desire to impress others or because you seek something in return; serve them because you want to serve, with a sincere and humble heart. In *chado*, the finest tea is not served by the host who constructs a tea room of gold and gilt. The most important ingredient, as with any meal, is the love put into it by the maker.

Kokoro ire

A story involving Japan's most famous tea master, Sen Rikyu (1522–1591), illustrates this point. It tells of a tea grower who once invited the great master to have tea.

Overwhelmed with joy at Rikyu's acceptance, the tea grower led him to the tearoom and served tea to Rikyu himself. However, in his excitement his hand trembled and he performed badly, dropping the tea scoop and

knocking the tea whisk over. The other guests, disciples of
Rikyu, snickered at the tea grower's manner of making
tea, but Rikyu was moved to say, "It was the finest."
    On the way home, one of the disciples asked Rikyu,
"Why were you so impressed by such a shameful
performance?" Rikyu answered, "This man did not
invite me with the idea of showing off his skill. He
simply wanted to serve me tea with his whole heart. He
devoted himself completely to making a bowl of tea for
me, not worrying about errors. I was struck by that
sincerity."

This is the route to higher realization in zen: To give for the sheer pleasure of giving. Sometimes we think a relationship requires lots of money, a fancy house, or lavish gifts. But the spirit of *kokoro ire*—the inclusion of one's whole heart— reminds us that nothing is more important than the love we show the people we're with. Every person is a manifestation of the divine spirit; thus, to be wholeheartedly with someone shows respect not only for that person, but for the great God-force that enlivens all things.

Sometimes people give out of a sense of duty or insecurity. Sex should not be a chore. If you're making love while thinking about the laundry or what you have to do at work tomorrow, your mind and body aren't connected. A halfhearted effort is not worth giving in anything. *Do not trudge along your path.* If you find your feet dragging, you're on the wrong path.

In turn, do not give out of an ego-driven desire to prove something in bed. So much of the advice on improving our sex lives focuses on technique—contortionist sexual positions, how to hit the G-spot, 101 ways to kiss. No matter how technically good a lover is, unless the heart is in it, the sex will soon feel empty, like a play by actors who are going through the motions. The *spirit* of lovemaking has to be there first—the spirit of giving. From that spirit, the technique follows.

Likewise, avoid giving over-earnestly. Good sex does not result from trying too hard. Just settle back and don't rush. As Rikyu says of *chado,*

> *It is good for the host and guest to try their best, and in consequence to satisfy each other. However, it is not good for them to aim for the goal of satisfaction from the beginning.*

All it takes to be a good lover is a giving heart. If the technique is clumsy, teach each other. It won't stay clumsy for long.

Do not make a big show of your giving, either, because that invites feelings of indebtedness or reciprocity. "Do good work in secret," the masters say. This is the Japanese concept of *toku*, which translates as "virtue," but in practice means "unrewarded good deed." *Toku* is like the love we shower on a newborn baby. As the baby grows, it knows nothing of our sacrifices; it just knows that it is happy. Therein lies our reward. Give to those you love in ways they'll never know, and you elevate the collective spirit of humanity.

Toku

There is no need to worry about getting something back, because when two lovers engage in intercourse, giving and receiving become the same thing. One lover is inside the other. The distinction between giving and getting is meaningless. In the words of the romantic philosopher Kahlil Gibran (1883–1931),

> *It is the pleasure of the bee to gather honey of the flower, but it is also the pleasure of the flower to yield its honey to the bee. For to the bee a flower is a fountain of life and to the flower a bee is a messenger of love, and to both, bee and flower, the giving and the receiving of pleasure is a need and an ecstasy.*

When you're truly one with everything, it doesn't matter what you give away, because you've still got everything. You can give freely from your heart, because the contents of your heart can never be exhausted. Zen masters say, "With sufficient depth, spring will amply supply stream." Whatever we give away, we will always feel replenished, because the source of our giving is boundless.

It is the wellspring of love.

the way to zen sex

do something good for your lover in secret,
something he or she might not even notice.

never tell a soul.

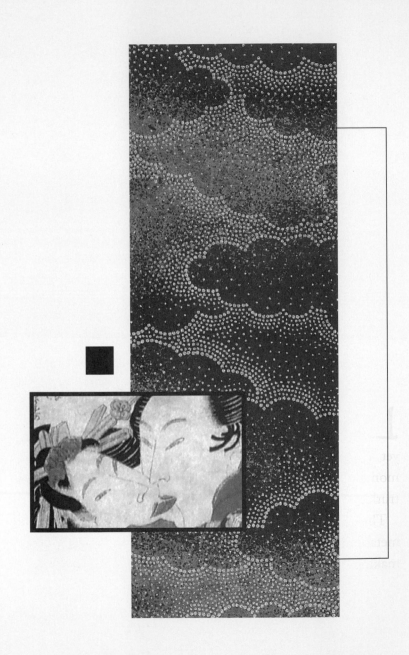

the way of clouds

Open your hand,
it becomes a cloud;
turn it over, rain.
—Zen saying

L ook at a cloud and you see something there, and yet not there. You can behold it, but not touch it. It has a form, yet is formless. In zen, we are all like clouds—here one moment, gone the next. The Way of Clouds is to know this truth and apply its spirit in lovemaking.

The ancient poets of China and Japan used "cloud-rain" as a metaphor for sex. To them, cloud-rain symbolized the heavens making love to the earth. Ikkyu used the imagery often:

Beautiful women's "cloud-rain" creates love's deeper rivers.
The pavilion girl and this old zen priest sing upstairs.

In Japan, wandering monks are called *unsui*—literally, "cloud and water"—as a reminder to be always floating and flowing. Ikkyu himself took the moniker Kyoun, or "Crazy Cloud," to describe his eccentric, non-conformist style of zen. (In Japan, the word *kyo* has connotations of bravery and high intention, of living outside the rules in order to retain the spirit of the rules.) He called his collected poems the "Crazy Cloud Anthology."

雲水

Unsui

My life has been devoted to love play;
I've no regrets about being tangled in red thread from head to foot,
Nor am I ashamed to have spent my days as a Crazy Cloud.

To be as a cloud in the bedroom, Ikkyu believed, exhibited the highest level of sexual artistry—making love light and free, completely in the here and now. He rhapsodized of his lover,

her mouth played with my cock
the way a cloud plays with the sky

The Way of Clouds is to acknowledge life's ephemeral nature and thus infuse one's lovemaking with immediacy. Life is short. We exist in but one pause. While we're here, make love like there's no tomorrow, because in zen, there *is* no tomorrow, only now. Says Ikkyu,

One short pause between
The leaky road here and
The never-leaking Way there:
If it rains, let it rain!
If it storms, let it storm!

Like clouds, we all assume different shapes in this life: thin, thick, wispy, fluffy, rolling, ominous, roiling. Know the spirit of the majestic cloud that covers a vast expanse of sea with its shadow; the misting cloud that kisses the valley with a sun shower; the thundercloud that pours hard rain down on the mountains. All these are the Way of Clouds.

No clouds, no rain.

No rain, no rainbows.

t h e w a y t o z e n s e x

lie back on the grass and watch the clouds overhead
as your lover licks and kisses you.

let it rain.

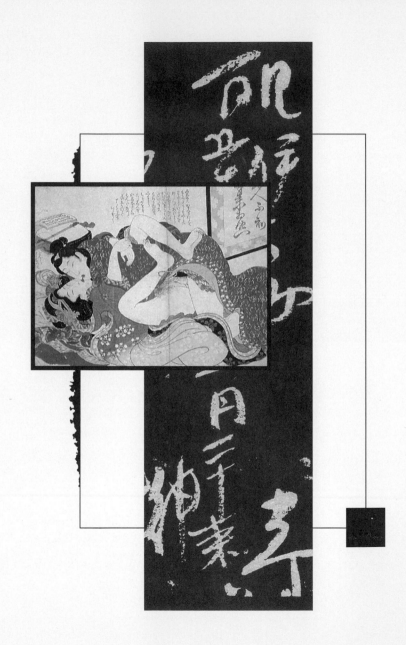

the way of union

you me when I think really think about it
are the same
—Ikkyu

In much of the world's mythology, the longing for sexual union is a longing for completeness. According to the Greek legend related by Aristophanes in Plato's *Symposium*, the gods split creatures in two so that each half feels incomplete without the other. The life that ensues is a process of searching for the perfect partner to make us whole.

In contrast, zen philosophy teaches that we are all inherently complete, just as we are. We need only awaken to that fact. "You have your own treasure-house," says the zen master Baso

(709–788). "Why do you search outside?" In this view, sex is not so much two halves moving toward completion as two wholes within a larger whole.

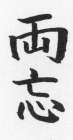

Ryo bo

The Way of Union is to recognize our individual wholeness, relate that to the universal whole, and *dissolve* that relationship as well. All things in this universe are united at the source, zen masters say; fundamentally, there is no separation between you and me, matter and space, heaven and earth. The masters say, *ryo bo*: Transcend the duality, or literally, "forget both in the heart."

At the same time, however, zen masters advise us—in typically paradoxical fashion—to revel in the variety of the divine. Relish the fact that there is more than one kind of relationship, more than one kind of love, more than one way to love someone. Just remember that in the end, all forms of love stem from the same source. "The One has many manifestations," they say, "and the Many have one essence."

The Way of Union is to express the principle of the One in our lovemaking and everything else we do. When two lovers realize this principle together, they create a whole greater than the sum of its parts. A transcendent element appears—a realization of the divine spirit coursing through us all. When we achieve that realization, it permeates all our daily activities, and the separate moments of our lives begin to form a seamless whole. Says Ikkyu,

> *for us no difference between reading eating singing*
> *making love not one thing or the other*

Too much of the time we live out of sync with ourselves, with mind, body, and spirit going in different directions. Zen challenges us to unify ourselves within and without—to live as one within the One. Penetrate deeply enough, the masters say, and find that point of unity where all senses converge. "To understand intimately," says the zen master Mumon, "one should see sound."

This is the beginner's mind, the mind of one newly born. Making love this way, sex becomes pure sensation—the touch, the taste, the cry of our lover all experienced as one. We are at one with ourselves, with our lover, and with the divine spirit. In this state, Ikkyu says,

> *you can't be anyone but you*
> *therefore you are that Other one you love*

Let the Way of Union remind us of the inextricable link between ourselves and the Other; that through all prejudice, hatred, divorce, and division, we are born of the same Great Mother and share a nameless last name.

Lovers of the world, unite.

the way to zen sex

finish making love.

stay locked with your partner for an extra moment.

when you part, take the One with you.

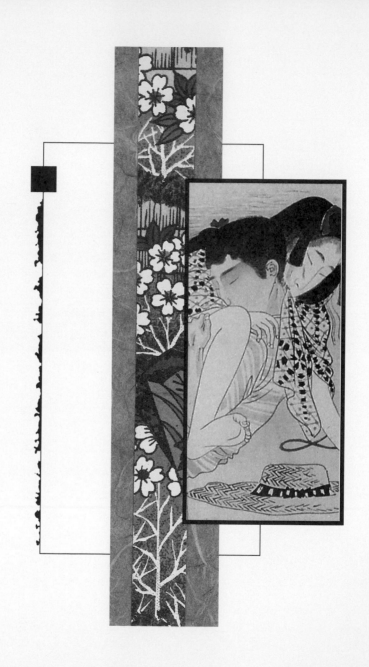

the way of release

Within your bedchamber, emotion for a torrent of poems.
Amid the flowers we sing and dance blissfully,
Sporting like mandarin ducks—
Our love play soars to heights unimagined.
—Ikkyu

The yin-yang principles of tension and release underlie every dramatic art form. The art of lovemaking is no exception. Play with yin and yang, and build that sexual tension to the breaking point. When the moment comes: *Let go.*

Great sex is sheer abandonment, letting go of inhibition and self-consciousness and giving in to the heat of the moment. In zen, every attachment must go—attachment to ego, self, body, possessions, this world, even to life itself. All this is symbolized in the moment of climax, when two lovers release and experience the feeling of transcendence. Through the Way of Release, we awaken to the God-power within us and glimpse our mortality and immortality at the same time.

Let go even of ideas about achieving orgasm. Sex should not be goal-oriented. Zen students who practice in order to achieve transcendence find that their very focus on transcendence prevents them from achieving it. It's like going after happiness as a goal. Happiness is not an end; it's a by-product of a life well lived. All that matters is the process—the *Way*. "The practice itself is enlightenment," the masters say. What results, results. Just do it, and let it come.

The French call orgasm *le petit mort*—"the little death." In that sense, every sexual release is an experience of the great Middle Way between life and death. Implicit in every sex act is our eventual death, as we move one step closer to the grave, but also the potential for new life, through procreation and the chance for enlightenment. As Ikkyu says,

> *Rinzai's disciples never got the zen message,*
> *But I, the Blind Donkey, know the truth:*
> *Love play can make you immortal.*

The route to that immortality is through letting go—or, in the vernacular of zen, through "emptying." Empty your cup, the masters say—completely. Don't hold on to a thing. Zen lore is replete with lessons about letting go. One of the most famous tells of an incident involving the zen master Tanzan and his disciple Ekido.

On a rainy day, the two men came upon a pretty woman looking to cross a muddy road. "Allow me," said Tanzan. Without hesitating, he lifted the woman in his arms and carried her across the street.

Ekido began brooding. That evening, he approached his master. "As monks, we've taken strict ascetic vows," he said. "We're not supposed to touch the opposite sex. How could you pick that woman up!?"

"I put the woman down at the side of the road," Tanzan said. "Are you still carrying her?"

In Tanzan's thinking, Ekido had failed to let go on several counts. He had clung to the rules and strictures of his practice, letting them regulate his actions instead of guide them. He had become obsessed with a pretty woman. And he could not let go of his anger toward his teacher. Meanwhile, Tanzan acted naturally and spontaneously in the flow of life. On his path of zen, a woman looking to cross the road had appeared, and he had helped her. When he put her down, he continued on his path and moved on. Like Ikkyu the Crazy Cloud, Tanzan transcended the rules of his station and, in so doing, stayed true to their intent. He knew how and when to let go.

So many of us cling to things in life that keep us from growing—a stale job, an unrequited love, bachelorhood, a pipe dream—when the time has come to let go and move on. We latch on to stations in life like we do our cherished possessions. "Living in the world yet not forming attachments to the dust of the world is the way of a true zen student," says the master Zengetsu.

This is much easier said than done, even on the highest levels of zen. Near the end of his life, Ikkyu says he simply can't let go of his sexual appetites:

> It's too difficult to stop being aware of the fair sex;
> Though my hair is snow-white, desires still sing through
>   my body.
> I cannot control all the "weeds" that grow in my garden.

And yet, zen teaching admonishes even those teachers who cling. An exchange between the master Mu-nan (1602–1676) and his disciple Shoju (1642–1721) shows how, all the way to the last step of life, zen practice must continue:

*On his deathbed, Mu-nan called Shoju into his room.
"Here is a book," he told his pupil. "It has been passed
down from master to master for seven generations. I also
have added many points according to my understanding.
The book is very valuable, and I am giving it to you to
represent your successorship."*

*"If the book is such an important thing, you had better
keep it," Shoju said. But the master insisted and put it
in Shoju's hand.*

*Shoju accepted the book and laid it on the flaming
coals of the brazier.*

"What are you doing!" Mu-nan shouted.

"What are you saying!" Shoju replied.

As the zen masters say, when the student is ready, the teacher
appears. In the end, Shoju became teacher to his master. Let
go, Shoju said. Nothing material lasts forever—not this book,
not this body.

We implicitly realize Shoju's lesson with each "little death" of
sexual release—*le petit mort,* an acknowledgment of life's
impermanence. This is the climax of all life: the moment of
death. The Way of Release reminds us that, in letting go
through sex, we must similarly let go in all of life. Empty your-

self of everything and you will be filled by the very source of your being: Love, endless and inexhaustible.

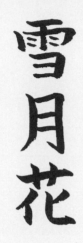

A three-word zen poem, *Setsu getsu ka*, expresses the Way of Release through the symbols of nature. It says simply, "Snow, moon, flower." The snow symbolizes winter and the season of decline—the "little death" implicit in the moment of sexual release. The moon symbolizes the monthly cycles of a woman and fertility. The flower symbolizes the spring, the season of new birth. Distilled into three words, "Snow, moon, flower" transmits the whole cycle of life and love.

Setsu getsu ka

In time, the flower, too, will fade and fall from the bush.

Such is the Way of Release.

t h e   w a y   t o   z e n   s e x

at the moment of climax, release all sexual tension.

where does it go?

follow it.

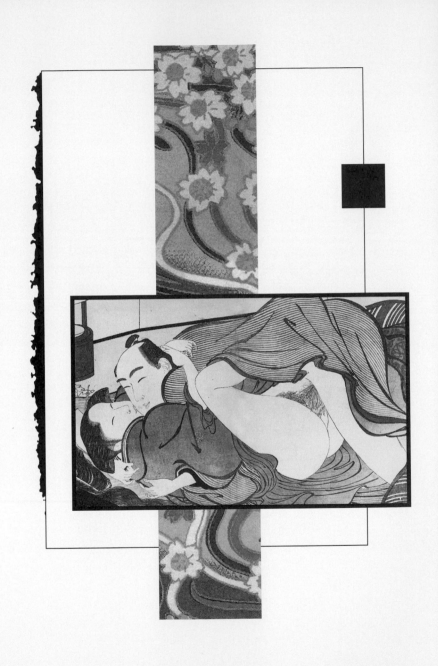

the way of creation

The lovemaking between the father and mother
produces the spark of life.
—Ikkyu

The Japanese have a saying, *Hotoke tsukutte tamashii irezu*: "Buddha's image is made but the spirit has not been put in." There's a certain soul that has to go into the making of something, that quality of *kokoro ire*, inclusion of the heart's spirit. We can carve a wooden Buddha, craft a table and chair, make a car, make money, or make music. But how much of ourselves do we put into the making? Whatever we set out to make, we should make as well as we can. To do otherwise is spiritless.

The Way of Creation is to make love.

What greater thing to make in this world than love? Put the spirit of Buddha, the God-spirit in you, into loving your partner. Therein lies the true transcendent climax of sex, when we feel that higher power of love, the *life force*, manifest itself through us and we give ourselves over to it.

Through sex, we connect ourselves to the long line of creation. Our parents created us. Now we, as their creations, in turn create the next generation of creators. Whether we conceive children or not, sex connects us to that process. Says Ikkyu,

> *passion's red thread is infinite*
> *like the earth always under me*

Just *make love* in sex—that is, create love and make it manifest in the world. Do so, and the love will carry forward through generations. The most obvious way is in the creation of a child. So many children are born into this world unwanted, so many pregnancies aborted. Better to be fully present in the moment of lovemaking, aware of the *making*. What spirit is the sperm carrying in its release? What spirit the egg? Put the spirit of Buddha, the God-spirit in you, into the creation of a little Buddha, so as to create a new God-spirit in the world. Ikkyu, who fathered a love child with Lady Mori, wrote of his newborn daughter,

Even among beauties she is a precious pearl;
A little princess in this sorry world.
She is the inevitable result of true love,
And a zen master is no match for her!

Conceiving a child is not the only way to make love manifest in the world. There are plenty of lovers who will never have children, yet their God-spirit passes on through generations. The zen masters say that even after death, we can transmit a feeling of *nyo zai*: "As if one is still here."

Nyo zai

The people who have great influence in our lives—parents, family, friends, teachers, and strangers—live on through us even after death. In this way, they are "still here." Their teachings stay alive, their sacrifices continue to make a difference, because our contributions make a difference. The zen masters of lore, centuries dead, are "still here" through their teachings, challenging us to push forward.

Through the Way of Creation, we become aware of the love that's been given us by generations past and we pass that love—

that spark of creation at our core—on to succeeding generations. In this way, a single act of lovemaking ripples outward
into the surrounding world. As the people we touch in turn
spread it to others, all of humanity benefits. From one act of
love, ten thousand lives feel the blessing. When Lady Mori
touches her lover Ikkyu, it brings the master such happiness
that even his disciples benefit:

*it's her freedom I love when I'm sick she makes me hard
fingers lips rove everywhere bring my followers joy*

Love begets love. That is the Way of Creation. Like Lady
Mori, make the best love that you can—not with effort, but
with *freedom*. Be the vehicle that gives form to the formless
energy. Feel it flow through you toward others, so that they
may spread it to others as well.

When lovemaking generates more love, we're reminded of
the Buddha's great lesson, when he gathered his disciples for a
lecture and wordlessly held up a flower. Only one in the crowd,
Kasyapa, smiled to indicate he understood the teacher's message: The divine truth is here for all to share.

We can discover the truth anywhere—in a flower, a crow's
caw, or a single night of passion. The glory of creation abounds

and surrounds. No words can express the feeling; no painter can capture its magnificence. Like the Buddha twirling a flower before his disciples, there is nothing to say.

Just make love and watch the other smile.

the way to zen sex

remember who made you
and those before you
and those before them.

all those ancestors are within you,
stretching back to Creation.

years hence,
whom will you be within?

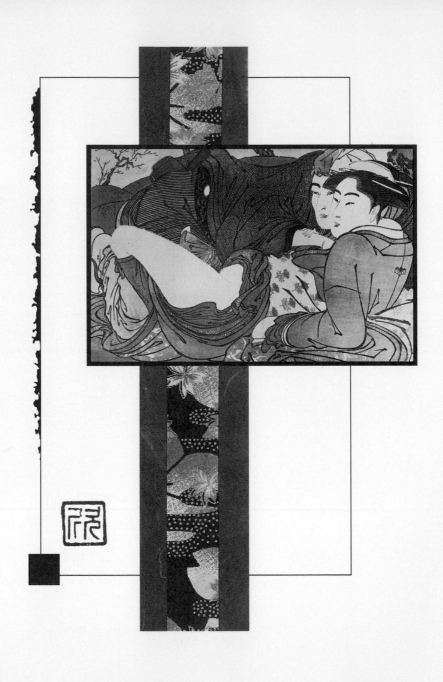

the way of birth and rebirth

before birth after birth
that's where you are now
—Ikkyu

When the poets of Asia use "cloud-rain" as a euphemism for lovemaking, they do so knowing that the image signifies the cycle of birth and rebirth: A cloud discharges rain, replenishing the waters; those waters vaporize and form new clouds, which in turn discharge new rain. This is the Way of Birth and Rebirth.

Making "cloud-rain" with our partner, we replenish each other; we shower new love on the world; we undergo our own spiritual rebirth. In this way, we reach that place of what the masters call "no coming and no going," or "not born and not dying." Sex becomes a means to transcend death. As Ikkyu says,

> it's logical: if you're not going anywhere
> any road is the right one

In sex, there is nowhere to go but right here, right now. All we need do is focus on this moment with our lover, without selfishness or thought. *I dedicate every pore to what's here*, is how Ikkyu puts it. The spiritual result of such lovemaking will ripple outward long after we die.

The Way of Birth and Rebirth is best described in one of zen's classic teachings, *Jugyu-Zu*, or "Ten Bull-Herding Pictures." The origins of the pictures date back centuries, although they are best known in a version created by the twelfth-century master Kakuan.

Kakuan said it was not enough for zen students to attain enlightenment. One had to know how to *live* with enlightenment. So he prescribed two things once enlightenment had been attained: To see the inherent beauty of all things, and to mingle among the people of the world so as to further the enlightenment of all beings. In the context of Zen Sex, that means we must see the divinity of every lover—not merely use someone to gratify ourselves, but connect with that person spiritually. And we must make love in such a way that it bestows bliss unto others—the kind of bliss a partner can take out of the bedroom and into the daily world.

In the stage immediately following enlightenment, Kakuan says, we must return "back to the source." He writes,

> *Returned to the origin, back at the source, all is*
> *completed.*
> *Nothing is better than suddenly being as blind and deaf.*
> *Inside his hermitage, he does not look out.*
> *Boundless, the river runs as it runs. Red bloom the*
> *flowers just as they bloom.*

When Kakuan says, "Inside his hermitage, he does not look out," he is describing an enlightened person gazing inward at the core of his being. But we've all experienced this stage at one time in our lives: in the womb. Finding enlightenment through sex is the same as being a newly conceived child; it is a return to the source from which all life comes. Those who make that return see that "boundless, the river runs as it runs," and "red bloom the flowers just as they bloom." Everything is as it should be. Flowing water flows. Flowers bloom anew. The beauty in every common thing and every living person radiates outward. Even "ordinary" sex becomes spiritual.

The highest expression of enlightenment, Kakuan says, is to live "in the world." He describes an enlightened person who moves among the people of the world with "bliss-bestowing hands":

> *Bare-chested and bare-footed he enters the market,*
> *Face streaked with dust and head covered with ashes,*
> *But a mighty laugh spreads from cheek to cheek.*
> *Without troubling himself to work miracles, suddenly*
> *   dead trees break into bloom.*

Who is this person?

You are. All of us are—at least we all were that person in the moment of our birth.

Without troubling himself to work miracles, a miracle occurs, for what is a newborn baby if not an everyday, commonplace miracle? *Face streaked with dust and head covered with ashes*, we enter as spirit into flesh, our mortal bodies reminding us of life's progression from ashes to ashes and dust to dust.

Each of us comes into this world as that baby, needing love and caring to survive. Not all of us get it. Others among us lose that sense of joy, the mighty laugh that spreads from cheek to cheek, as we grow older and bear the burdens of adulthood. But we can become that person once again—born again through spiritual sex. We have a choice to renew ourselves in spite of our past. Therein lies the key to our rebirth.

Through the Way of Birth and Rebirth, we bestow bliss with each act of lovemaking. Every night of passion becomes an opportunity to elevate the human spirit. Every child conceived becomes a manifestation of our love for humanity. Do not retreat from the world in your hermitage. Do not hide inside the bedroom, squirreled away with your lover. Make love, and take that love out into the world to make new love. Therein lies your birth and rebirth.

If we can pass the true spirit of lovemaking on to future generations, we will have done our duty. Let that be our legacy to the children of today, and to their children, so that long after we've gone and passed away, those who'll never know us can feel *nyo zai*: As if one is still there.

The one is you.

the way to zen sex

from a tiny seed and egg
you were born
given a name
nourished
schooled
to this complex self you are
reading these words
right now.

from this moment forward
make Love
reborn.

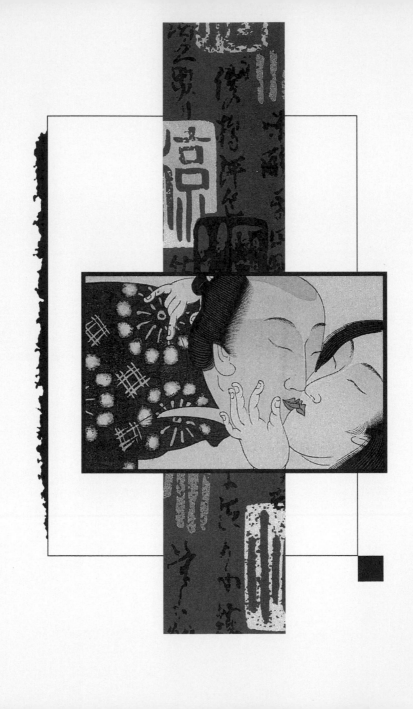

the way of making love

Return to the origin

Enter naked
Creator
Created

One sperm
One egg

One spirit
One sex

Revel in your body
Feel your surface
Touch each other freely
Live your love

Follow your lust to the source
Use your imagination
Wear what your lover likes
Play your favorite song
Go where the mood takes you
Show the mood in your eyes

Open the door
To your bedroom
To what lies beyond

Invite your lover in
Let yourself be taken

Relax in the tension
Put technique aside
Do not rush
Do not be afraid
Let love come

Give without thought of getting
Do it because you want to
Pour in every ounce of your heart and soul

Teach a new pleasure
Show what you want to do,
What you want done to you.
Don't try. Do.

Use your mouth
Everywhere, every way
Savor the taste
Breathe heavily
Fill the silence with cries, sighs, and moans

Vary your rhythm
Align your rhythm within and without
Go deeper
Let go

Frolic. Tumble.
Laugh and play

Be as a perfect mirror,
Reflecting the light from within

Under the moon
Under the sun
Make the first move

Gaze into your lover's eyes
See yourself
A cloud
Floating
Filled with rain

Make Love
Here
Now
Anywhere
One time, one meeting

Do it again

and again

and again

Fall together in blissful sleep,
Dreaming the dream of the dreamer dreaming.

Today is your birthday

Awaken

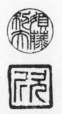

about the images

The images presented in this book are examples of the Japanese art form *shunga*, or "spring pictures," which flourished from the early seventeenth century through the late nineteenth century. *Shunga* served as illustrations for love novels, posters for the pleasure quarters, and instruction guides for young wives and newly married couples.

Many of the images here were graciously provided by Ronin Gallery, a New York–based dealer in Japanese artwork. The gallery notes that "virtually all the great masters of the era believed that designing good *shunga* was vital to their artistic stature and considered its production important to their full development as an artist." These masters included Kitagawa Utamaro (1753–1808), Katsushika Hokusai (1760–1849), and Kikugawa Eizan (1787–1867). To them, Ronin notes, "human sexuality was the apex of all organic cycles, and they delineated its features as precisely and tenderly as they would any aspect of the natural world."

For a more extensive history of *shunga*, visit the Ronin Gallery web site at www.japancollection.com or contact Ronin Gallery, 605 Madison Avenue, New York, NY 10022, e-mail: ronin@japancollection.com.

images
P. viii: Kitagawa Utamaro, c. 1788. Victoria and Albert Museum, London, Great Britain/Art Resource, NY.

P. x: Anonymous Meiji Period artist, c. 1890. Ronin Gallery, New York City.

P. 10: Attributed to Kikugawa Eizan, c. 1820. Ronin Gallery, New York City.

P. 12: Attributed to Katsushika Hokusai, c. 1820. Ronin Gallery, New York City.

P. 24: Isoda Koryusai, c. 1770. Victoria and Albert Museum, London, Great Britain/Art Resource, NY.

P. 32: Anonymous Meiji Period artist, c. 1890. Ronin Gallery, New York City.

P. 40: Attributed to Eizan, c. 1820. Ronin Gallery, New York City.

P. 48: Attributed to Utamaro, c. 1795. Ronin Gallery, New York City.

P. 56: Suzuki Harunobu, c. 1765. Art Resource, NY.

P. 64: Anonymous, c. 1930, owned by the author.

P. 72: Anonymous, c. 1930, owned by the author.

P. 74: Attributed to Hokusai, c. 1820. Ronin Gallery, New York City.

P. 82: Attributed to Harunobu, c. 1765. Ronin Gallery, New York City.

P. 92: Attributed to Koryusai, c. 1770. Ronin Gallery, New York City.

P. 98: Anonymous Meiji Period artist, c. 1900. Ronin Gallery, New York City.

P. 104: Attributed to Eizan, c. 1820. Ronin Gallery, New York City.

P. 112: Anonymous, c. 1930, owned by the author.

P. 120: Anonymous Meiji Period artist, c. 1890. Ronin Gallery, New York City.

P. 126: Attributed to Torii Kiyonage, c. 1780. Ronin Gallery, New York City.

P. 128: Anonymous, c. 1930, owned by the author.

P. 138: Attributed to Katsukawa Shuncho, c. 1790. Ronin Gallery, New York City.

P. 146: Attributed to Hokusai, c. 1820. Ronin Gallery, New York City.

P. 152: Attributed to Eizan, c. 1820. Ronin Gallery, New York City.

P. 158: Anonymous Meiji Period artist, c. 1900. Ronin Gallery, New York City.

P. 166: Utamaro, c. 1788. Victoria and Albert Museum, London, Great Britain/Art Resource, NY.

P. 174: Utamaro, c. 1788. Victoria and Albert Museum, London, Great Britain/Art Resource, NY.

P. 182: Anonymous, c. 1930, owned by the author.

note on sources

The Ikkyu poetry quoted in this book came primarily from two translations: Stephen Berg's *Crow With No Mouth: Ikkyu, 15th Century Zen Master* (Copper Canyon Press), and John Stevens' *Wild Ways: Zen Poems of Ikkyu* (Shambhala). Both are highly recommended.

For background on Ikkyu's life and times, I relied heavily upon Jon Etta Hastings Carter Covell's *Unravelling Zen's Red Thread: Ikkyu's Controversial Way* (Hollym International), a thorough piece of scholarship that has sadly fallen out of print. I also turned to John Stevens' biography of Ikkyu in *Zen Masters: A Maverick, a Master of Masters, and a Wandering Poet* (Kodansha International).

Among the many versions of the *Tao Te Ching*, I chose Ray Grigg's "zen translation" of the *New Lao Tzu* (Charles E. Tuttle) for the way it addresses the modern reader.

The list of common sexual fantasies I found at http://www.sexuality.org, a vast and informative resource on matters of human sexuality.

Other sources that proved vital to this book are listed in the Select Bibliography, but particular mention goes to Paul Reps' classic *Zen Flesh, Zen Bones* (Anchor) for its treasure trove of zen anecdotes, and Soshitsu Sen XV's out-of-print gem *Tea Life, Tea Mind* (Weatherhill) for its application to all human relations.

For more detailed notes on sources, visit the Zen Sex web site at www.zensex.org.

select bibliography

Berg, Stephen. *Crow With No Mouth: Ikkyu, 15th Century Zen Master.* Port Townsend, WA: Copper Canyon Press, 1989.

Campbell, Joseph, with Bill Moyers. *The Power of Myth.* New York: Doubleday, 1988.

Chopra, Deepak, ed. *The Love Poems of Rumi.* Trans. Deepak Chopra and Fereydoun Kia. New York: Harmony, 1998.

Cleary, Thomas, trans. *The Ecstasy of Enlightenment.* York Beach, ME: Samuel Weiser, 1998.

Covell, Jon Etta Hastings Carter. *Unraveling Zen's Red Thread: Ikkyu's Controversial Way.* Elizabeth, NJ: Hollym International, 1980.

Deng Ming-Dao. *365 Tao.* San Francisco: HarperSanFrancisco, 1992.

Faure, Bernard. *The Red Thread: Buddhist Approaches to Sexuality.* Princeton, NJ: Princeton Univ. Press, 1998.

Fields, Rick, and Brian Cutillo, trans. *The Turquoise Bee: The Lovesongs of the Sixth Dalai Lama.* San Francisco: HarperSanFrancisco, 1994.

Franck, Frederick. *Zen Seeing, Zen Drawing: Meditation in Action.* New York: Bantam Books, 1993.

Gibran, Kahlil. *The Prophet.* New York: Alfred A. Knopf, 1923.

Grigg, Ray. *The New Lao Tzu.* Rutland, VT: Charles E. Tuttle, 1995.

Hyams, Joe. *Zen in the Martial Arts*. New York: Bantam Books, 1979.

Miners, Scott, ed. *A Spiritual Approach to Male/Female Relations.* Wheaton, IL: Quest/Theosophical Publishing, 1984.

Musashi, Miyamoto. *The Book of Five Rings*. Trans. Nihon Services Corp. New York: Bantam Books, 1982.

Myokyo-ni, Venerable. *Gentling the Bull: The Ten Bull Pictures, a Spiritual Journey.* Boston: Charles E. Tuttle, 1988.

Osbon, Diane K., ed. *A Joseph Campbell Companion: Reflections on the Art of Living.* New York: HarperPerennial, 1991.

Reps, Paul. *Zen Flesh, Zen Bones*. New York: Anchor Books, 1961.

Sekida, Katsuki. *Two Zen Classics*. New York: Weatherhill, 1977.

The Shambhala Dictionary of Buddhism and Zen. Boston: Shambhala, 1991.

Shigematsu, Soiku, trans. *A Zen Forest: Sayings of the Masters*. New York: Weatherhill, 1981.

Shimano, Eido Tai, and Kogetsu Tani. *Zen Word, Zen Calligraphy.* Boston: Shambhala, 1990.

Soshitsu Sen XV. *Tea Life, Tea Mind*. New York: Weatherhill, 1979.

Stevens, John. *Zen Masters: A Maverick, a Master of Masters, and a Wandering Poet*. Tokyo: Kodansha International, 1999.

————, ed. and trans. *Wild Ways: Zen Poems of Ikkyu.* Boston: Shambhala, 1995.

Sudo, Philip Toshio. *Zen Computer: Mindfulness and the Machine.* New York: Simon & Schuster, 1999.

————. *Zen Guitar.* New York: Simon & Schuster, 1997.

Sun Tzu. *The Art of War.* Trans. Samuel B. Griffith. Oxford: Oxford Univ. Press, 1963.

acknowledgments

Loving thanks to:
My mother and father, who made love and brought me into the world;
My brothers, Rich and Paul, born of the same love;
My ancestors, who've shaped me and live on through me in ways I'll never know;

My friends and colleagues Herbert Buchsbaum and Steven Manning, who each in his own way gave birth to the idea for this book;
My angel of an agent, Laurie Fox, who turns dreams into reality;
My editor, Doug Abrams, who saw where the book was and guided me toward it.

Thanks also to:
Renee Sedliar, for steering the book through all its twists and turns;
C. M. Hardt, for the vital early reading and support;
May Egner, for all the design insights and support;
Salvatore Principato, for the photography and coming through when I really needed it;
Roni Neuer at Ronin Gallery for so generously providing the artwork.

And lastly, mostly, to:
Naomi, Keith, and Jonathan, without whose love this never would have been written;

and to Tracy—
for all the nights of "research";
for the bliss of sleeping next to you;
and the joy of awakening
by your side.

permissions

Grateful acknowledgment is given to the following for permission to include excerpts from previously published works as well as original material:

Poems from *Crow With No Mouth* © 1989 by Stephen Berg.
Reprinted by permission of Copper Canyon Press, Post Office Box 271,
Port Townsend, WA 98368

Wild Ways: Zen Poems of Ikkyu © 1995, translated and edited by John Stevens.
Reprinted by arrangement with Shambhala Publications, Inc., Boston.

New Lao Tzu © 1995, by Ray Grigg. Reprinted by permission of
Charles E. Tuttle Co., Inc., of Boston, Massachusetts, and Tokyo, Japan.

Excerpts, as submitted from *The Turquoise Bee: Love Poems of the Sixth Dalai
Lama,* © 1994 by Rick Fields, Brian Cutillo and Mayumi Oda. Translated by
Rick Fields, Brian Cutillo, and Mayumi Oda. Reprinted by permission of
HarperCollins Publishers, Inc.

author contact

Visit the Zen Sex web site at:
www.zensex.org

Read material from the author's other works at:
www.zenguitar.com
www.zencomputer.com